THIS BOOK BELONGS TO

_____

HUMAN BODY ANATOMY COLORING

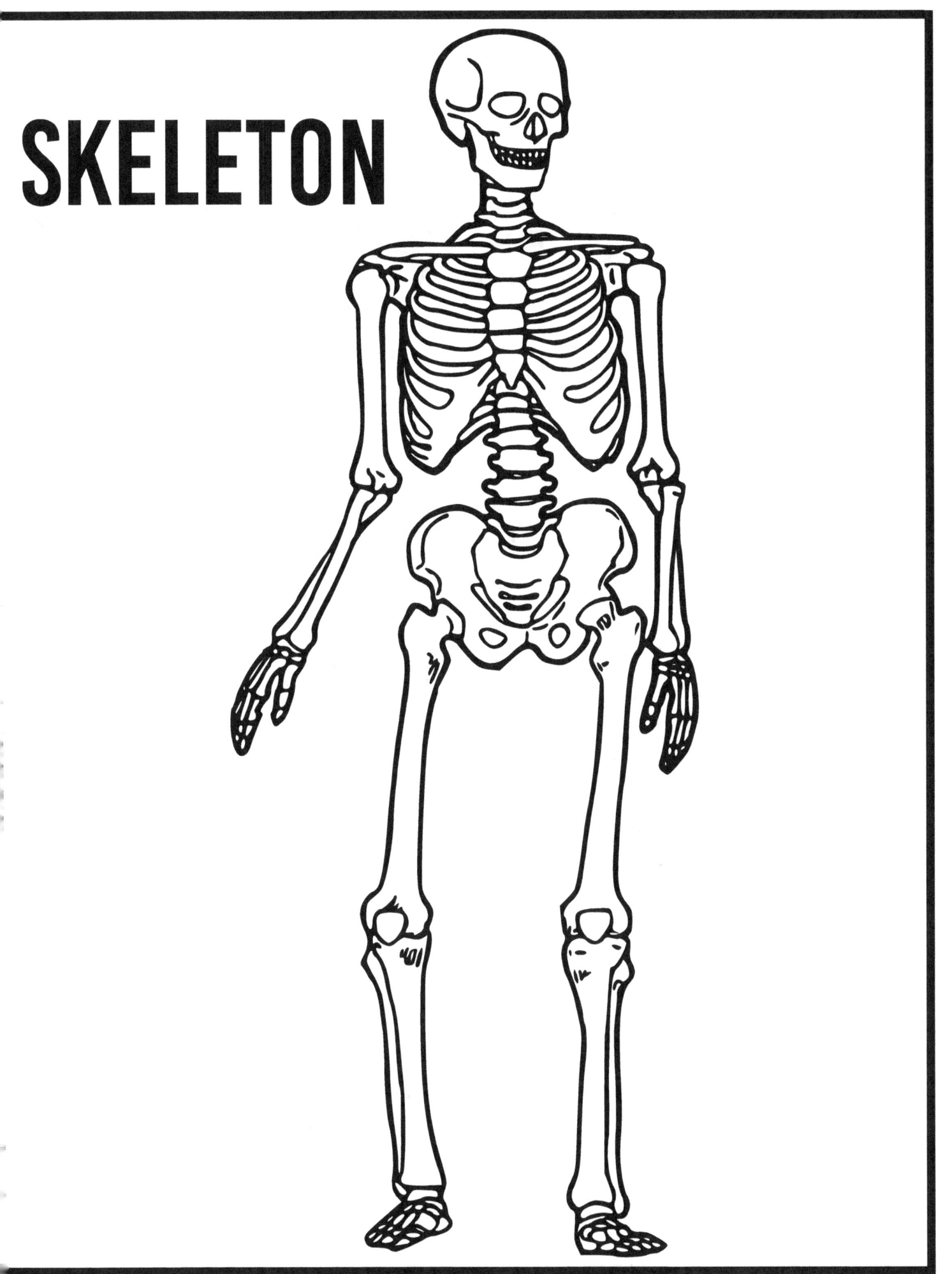

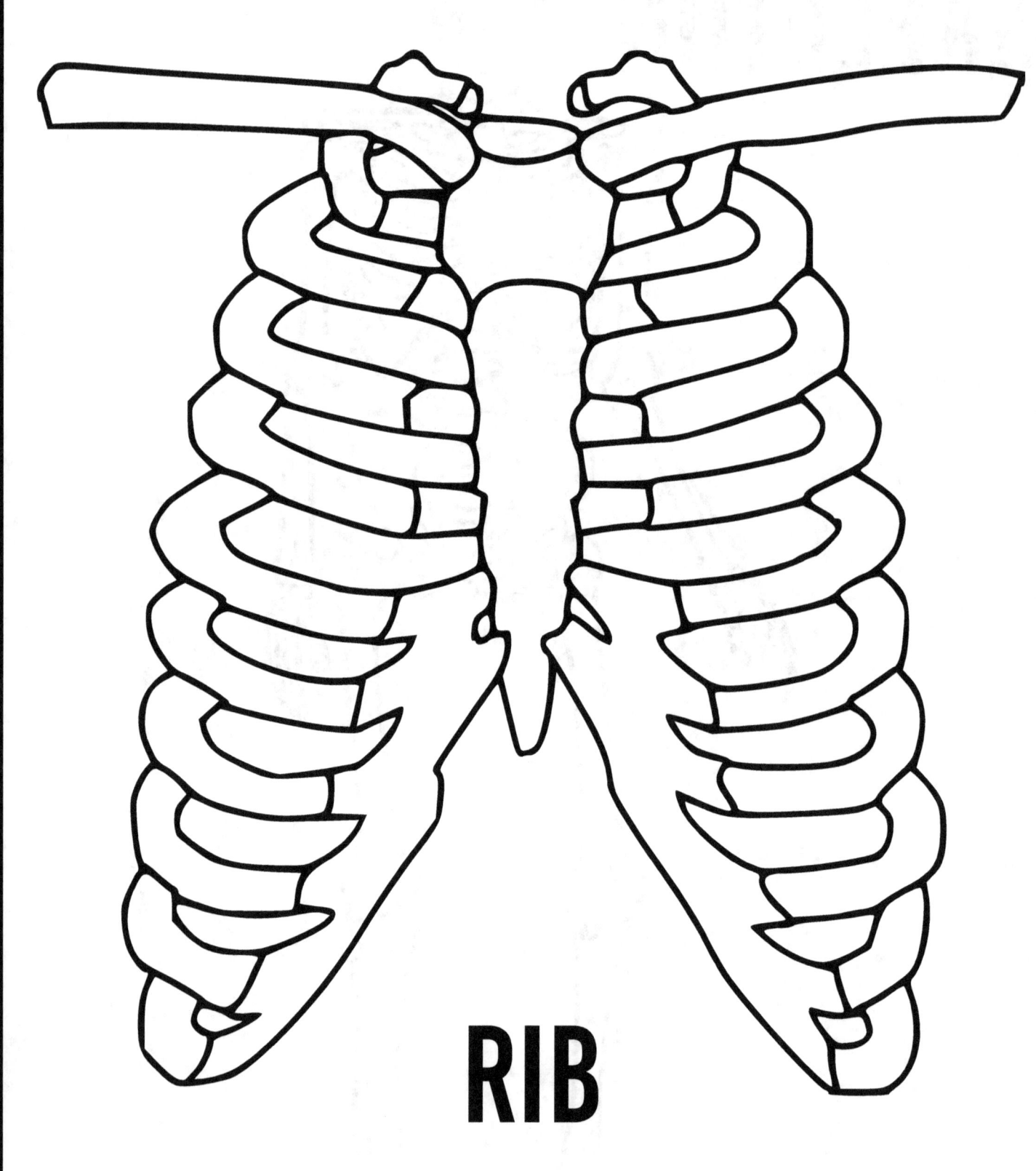

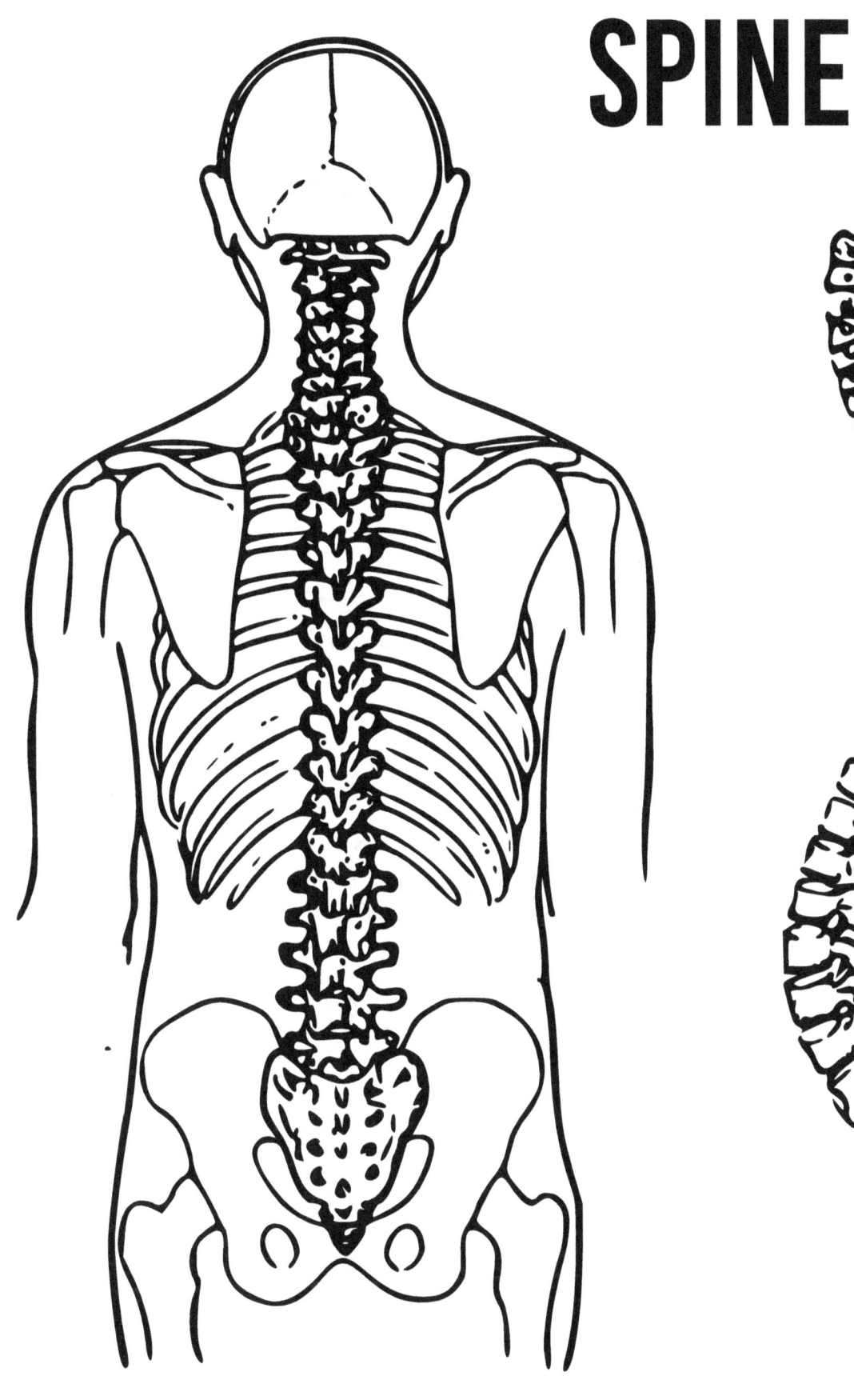

FOOT

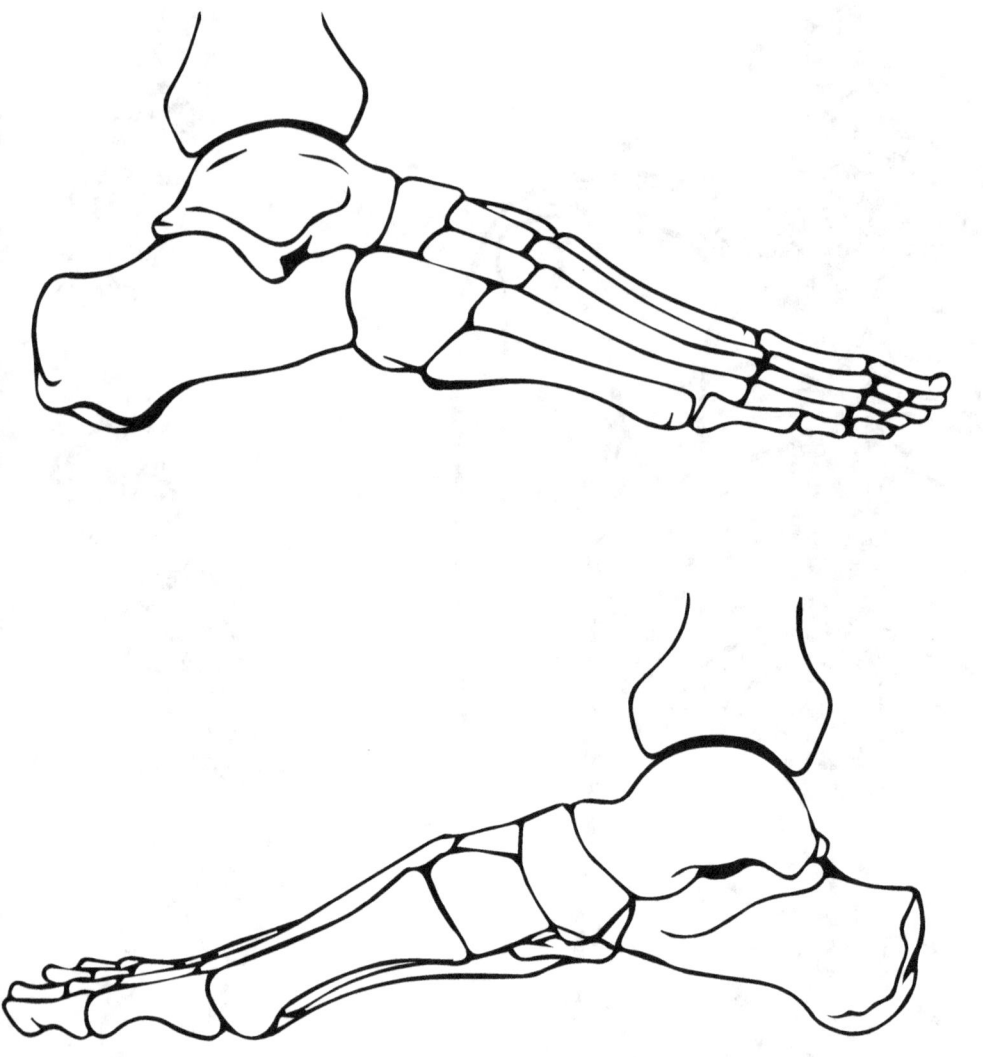
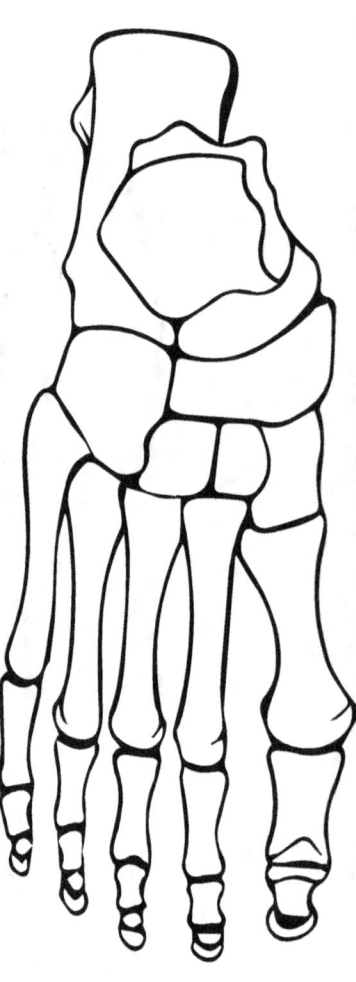

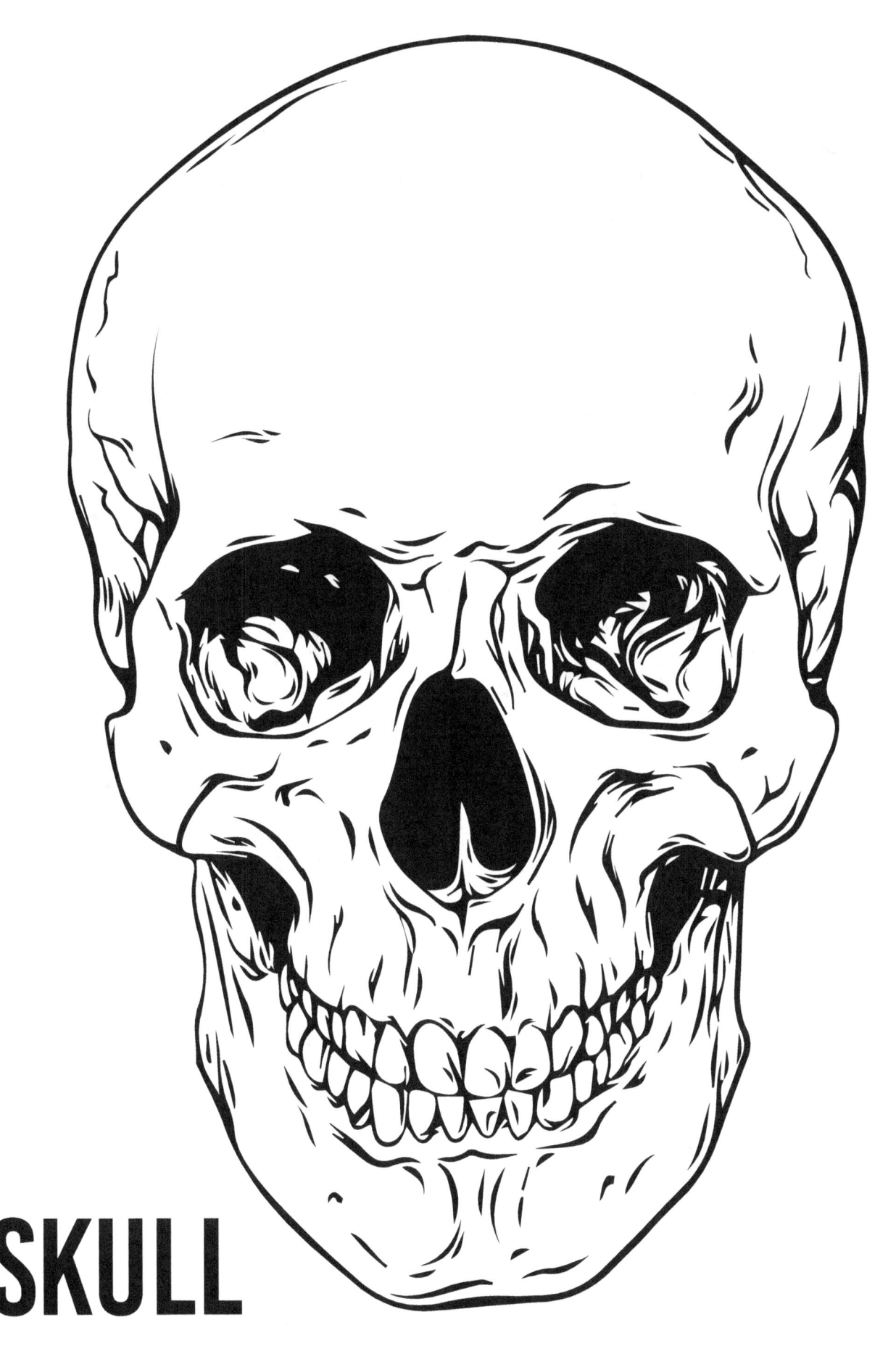

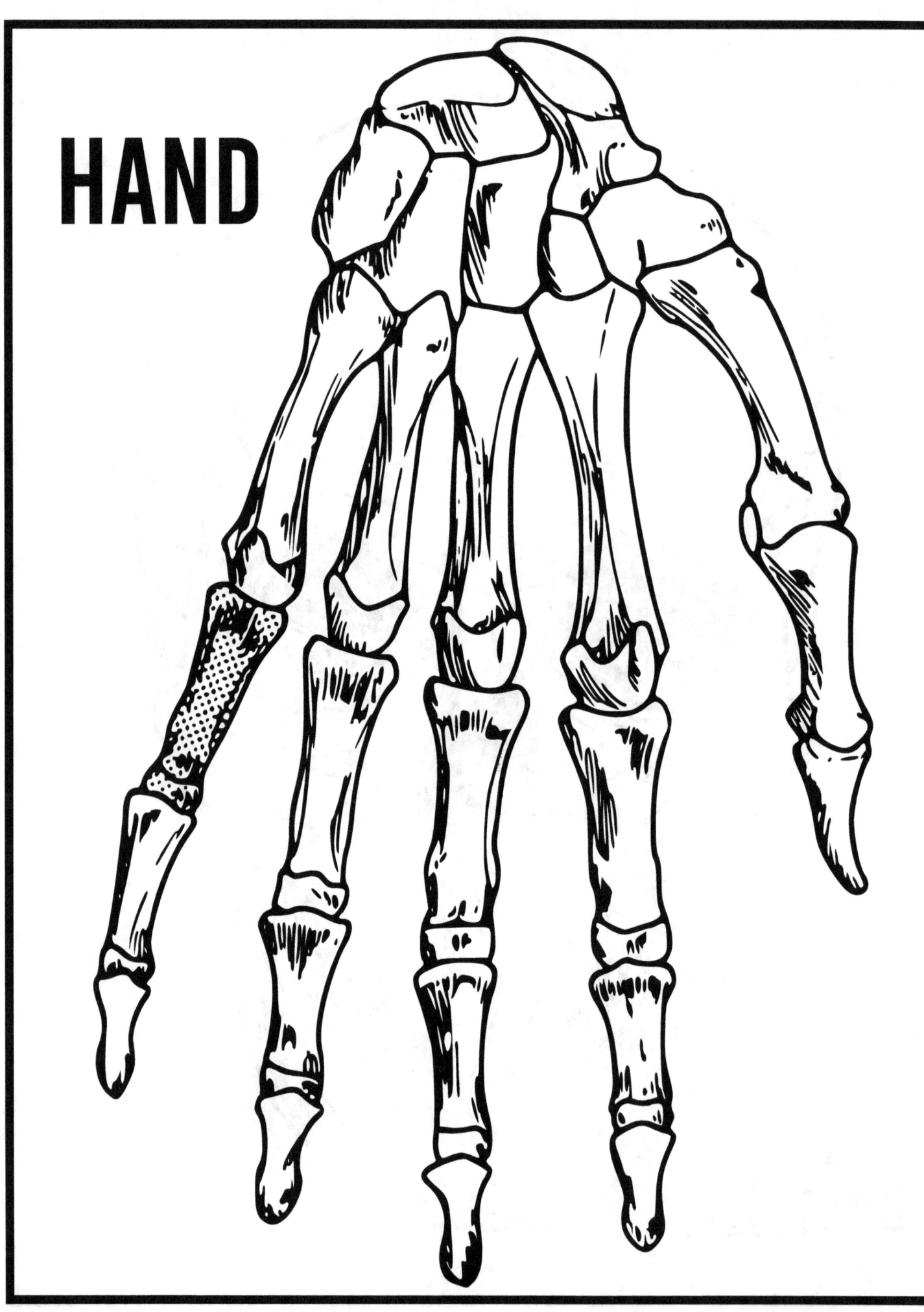

PELVIS

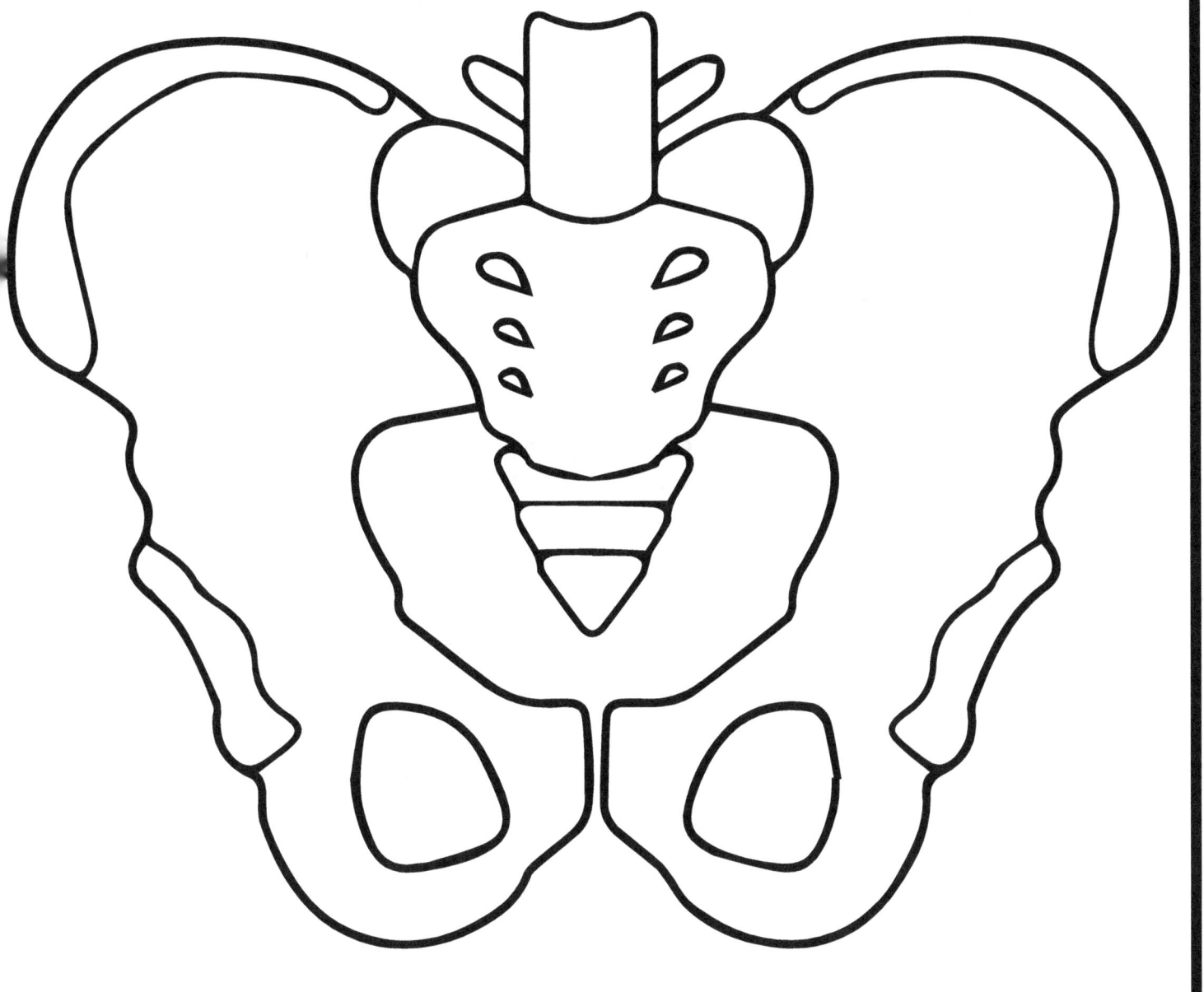

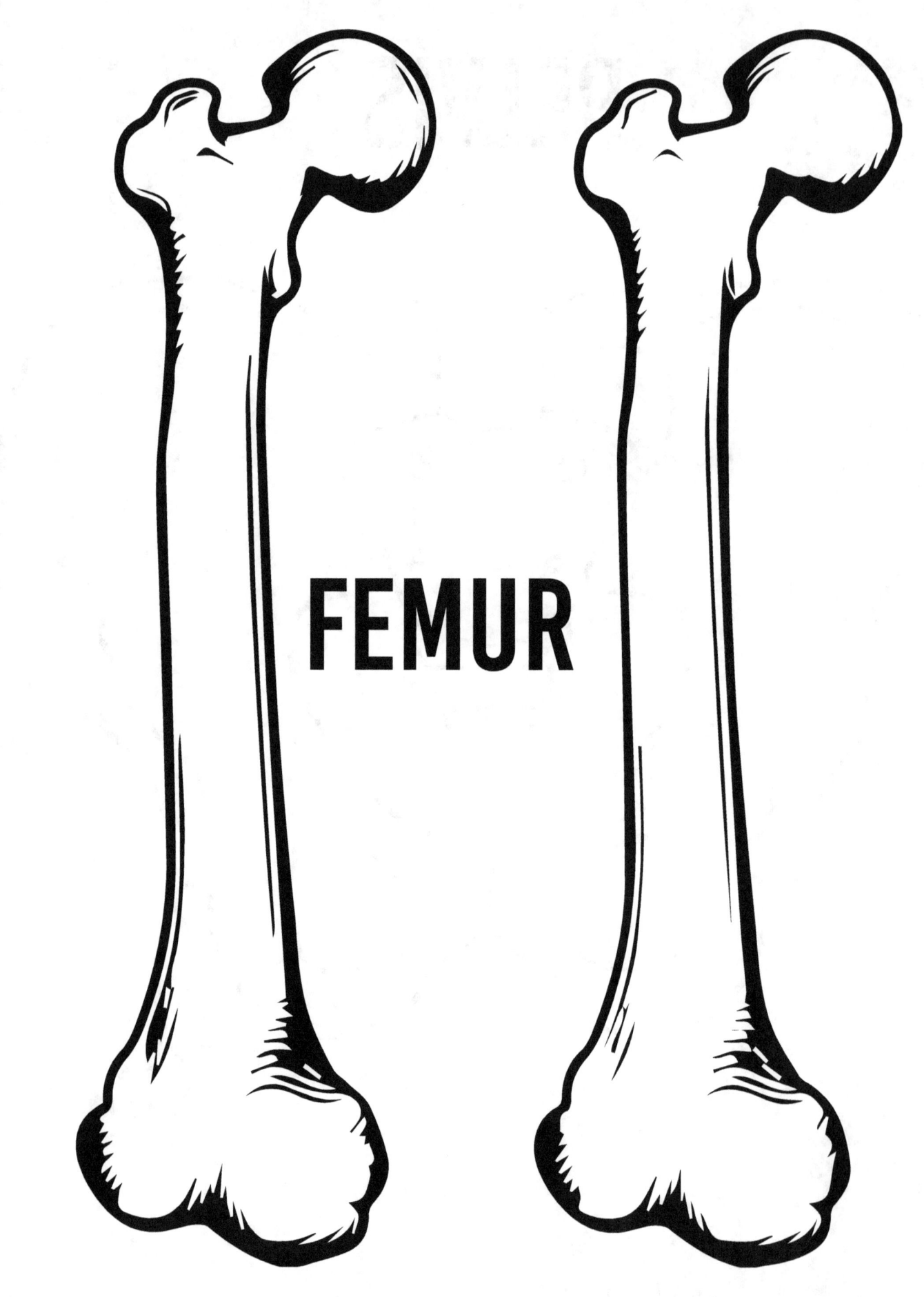

BRAIN

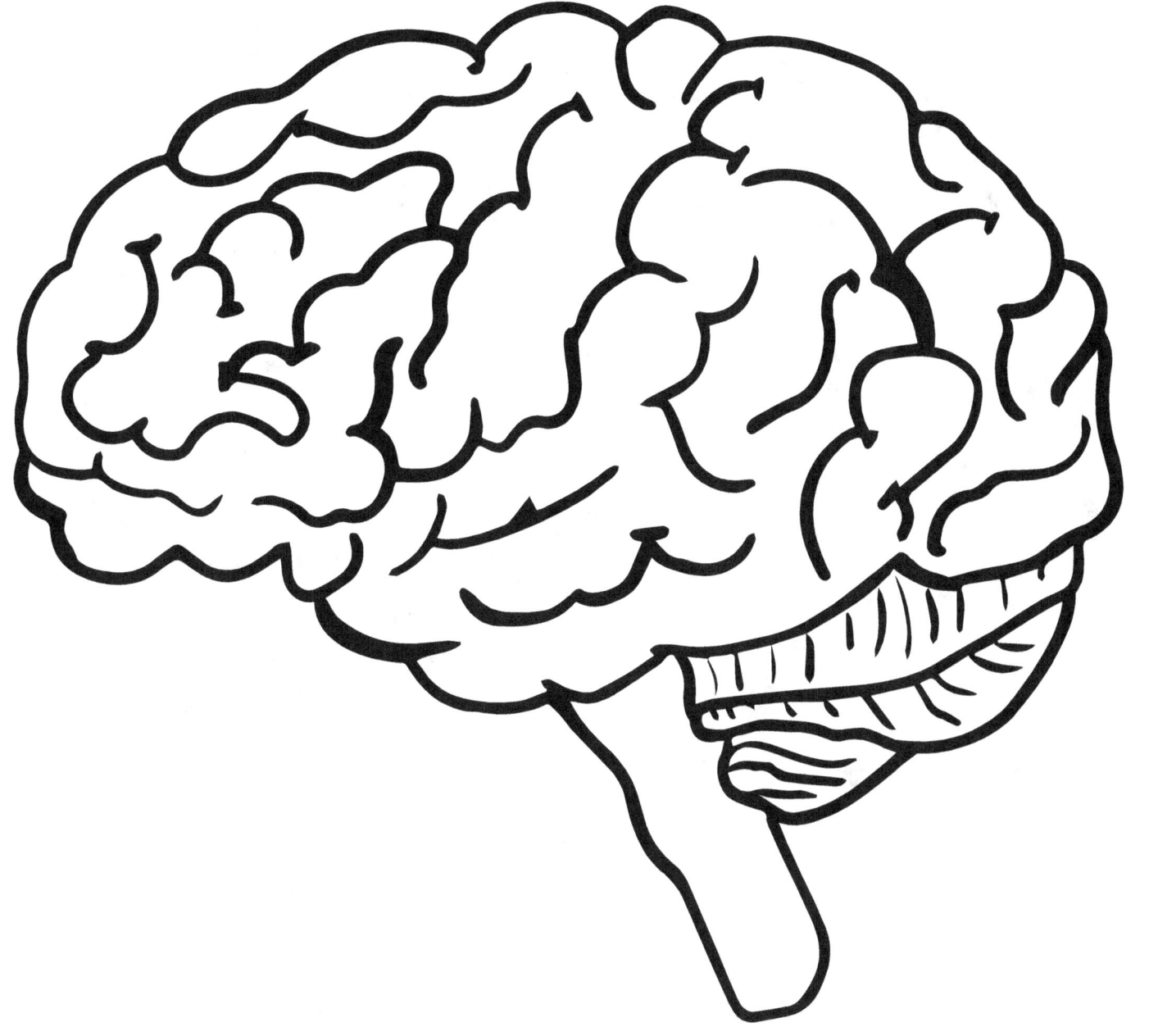

TOP VIEW

SPLEEN

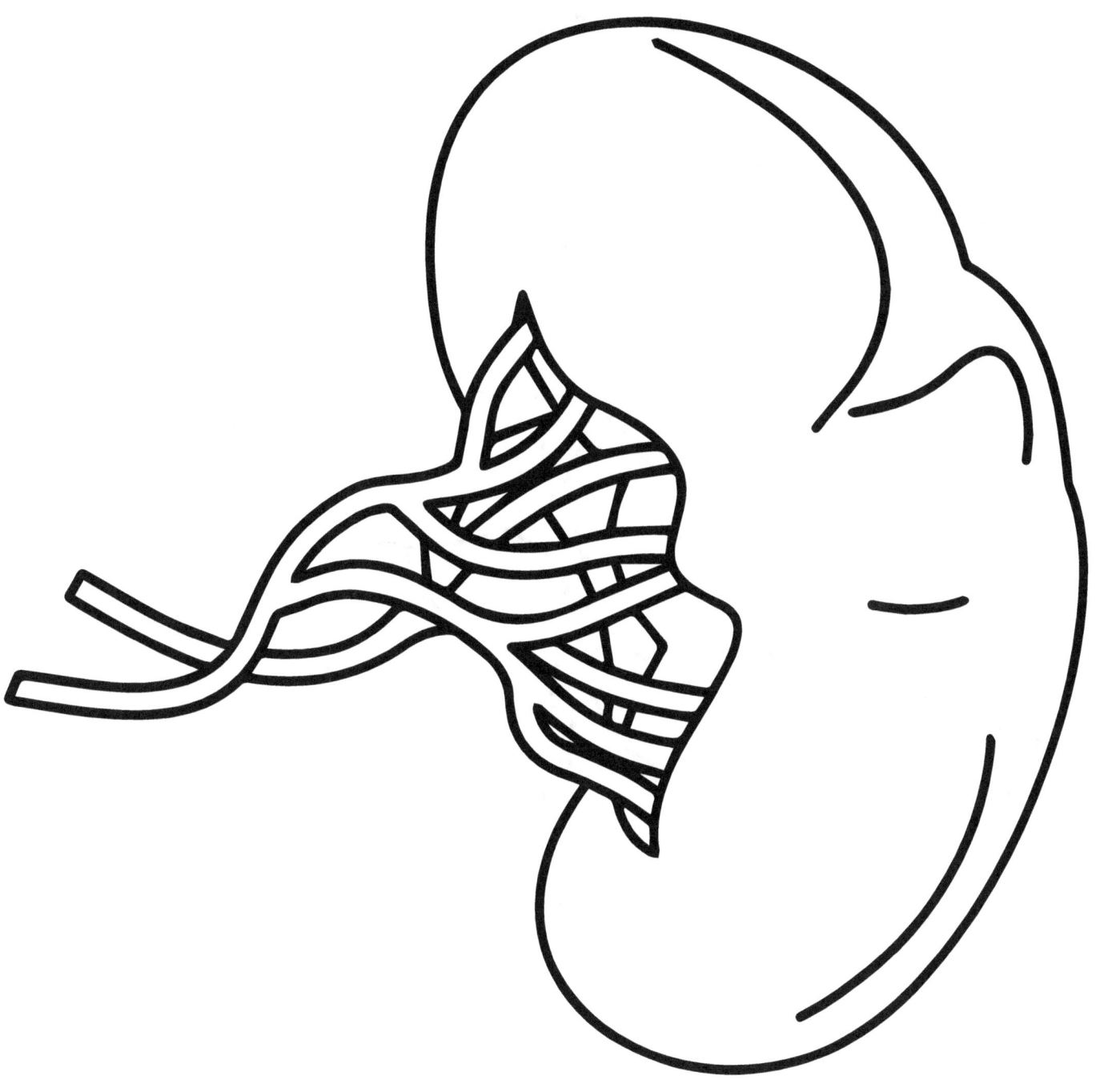

LIVER

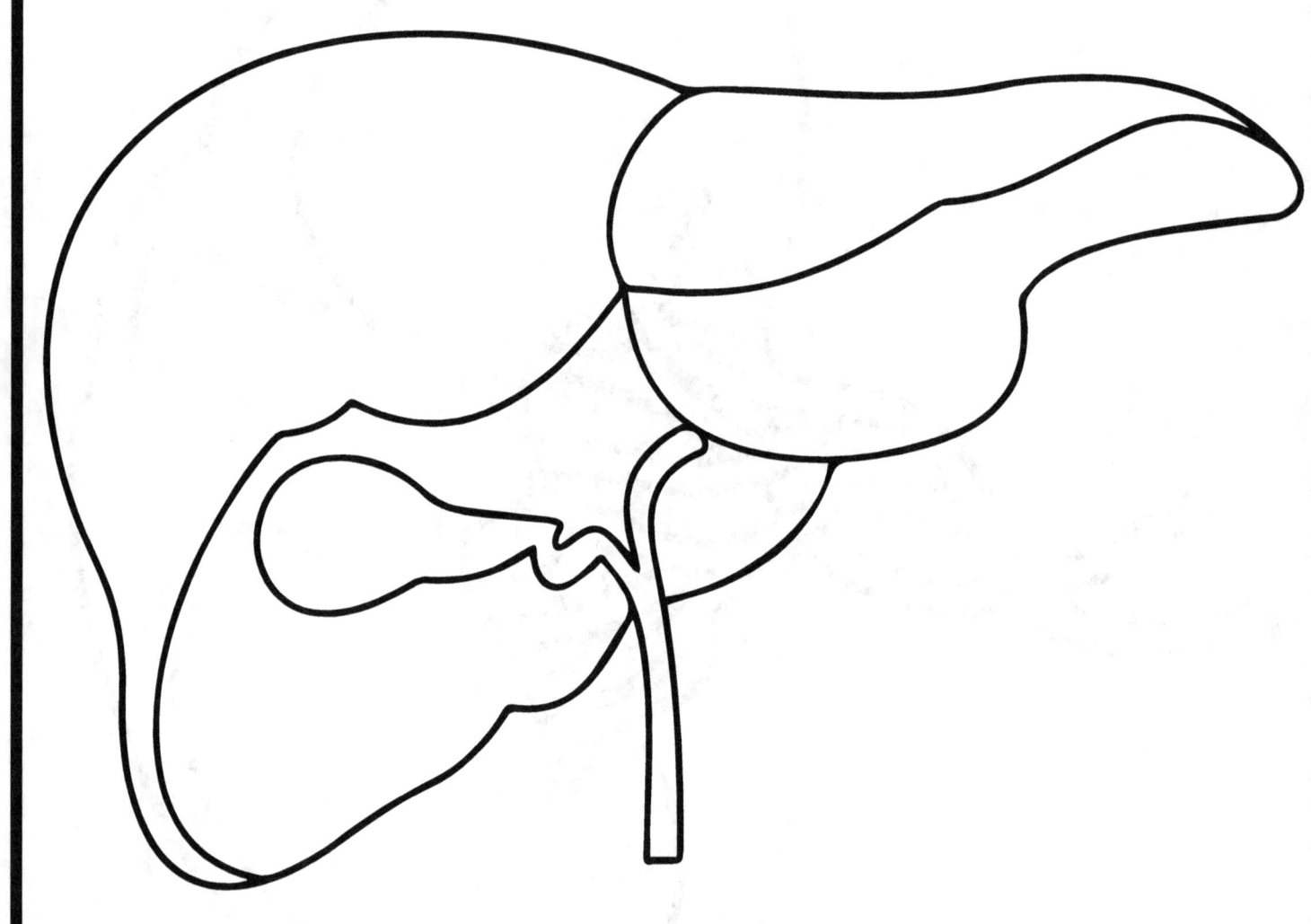

LIVER (CROSS SELECTION)

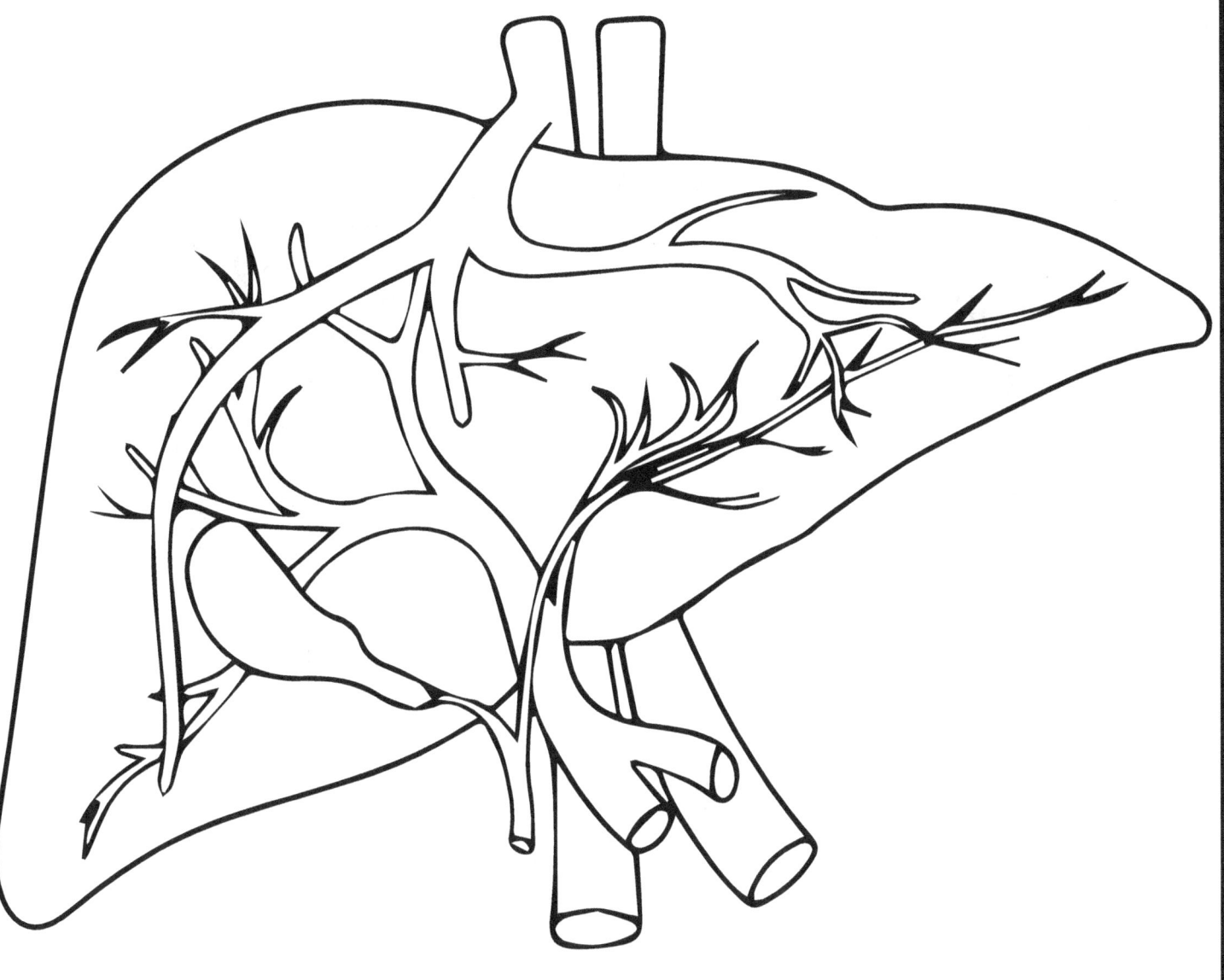

BLADDER

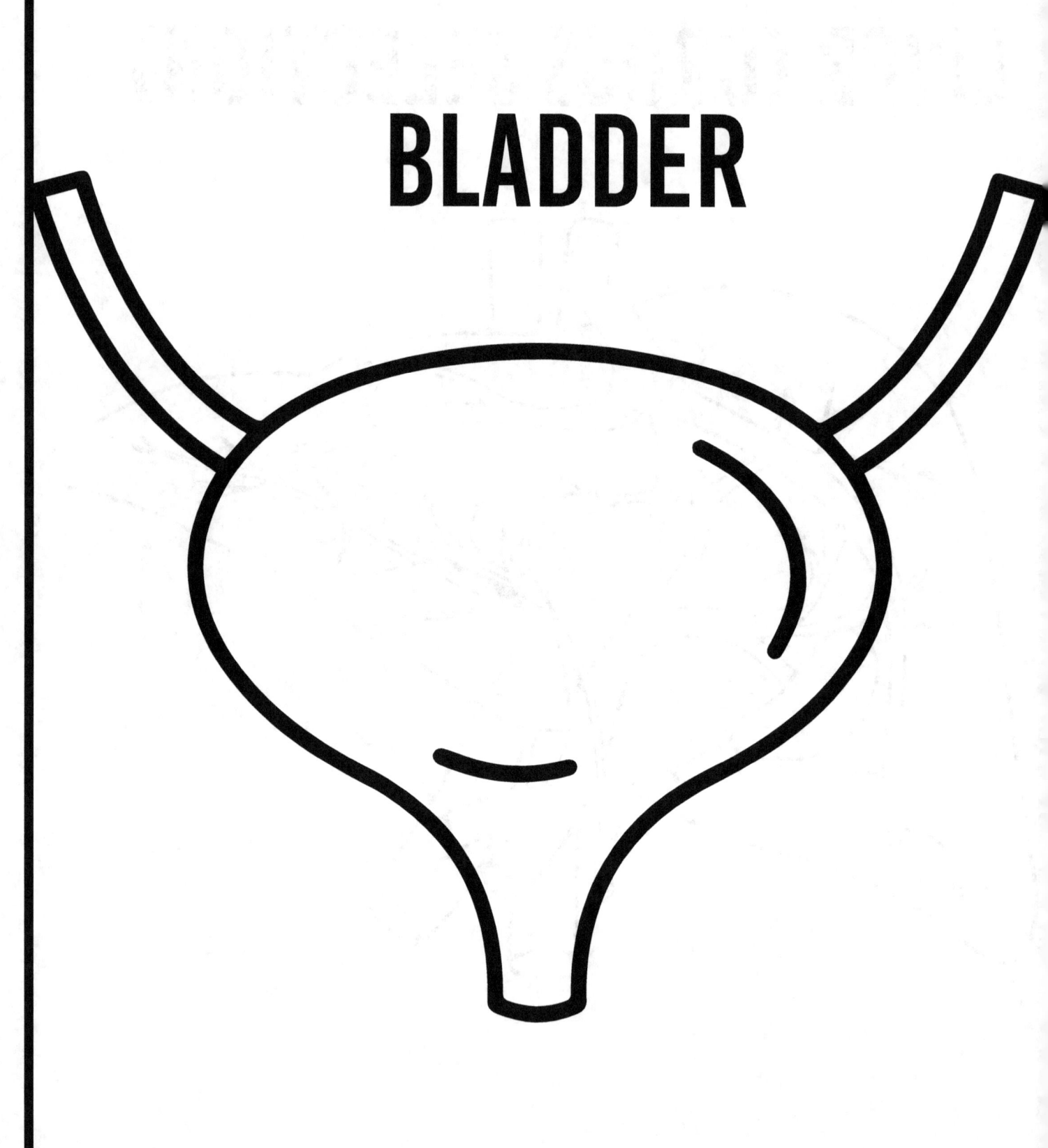

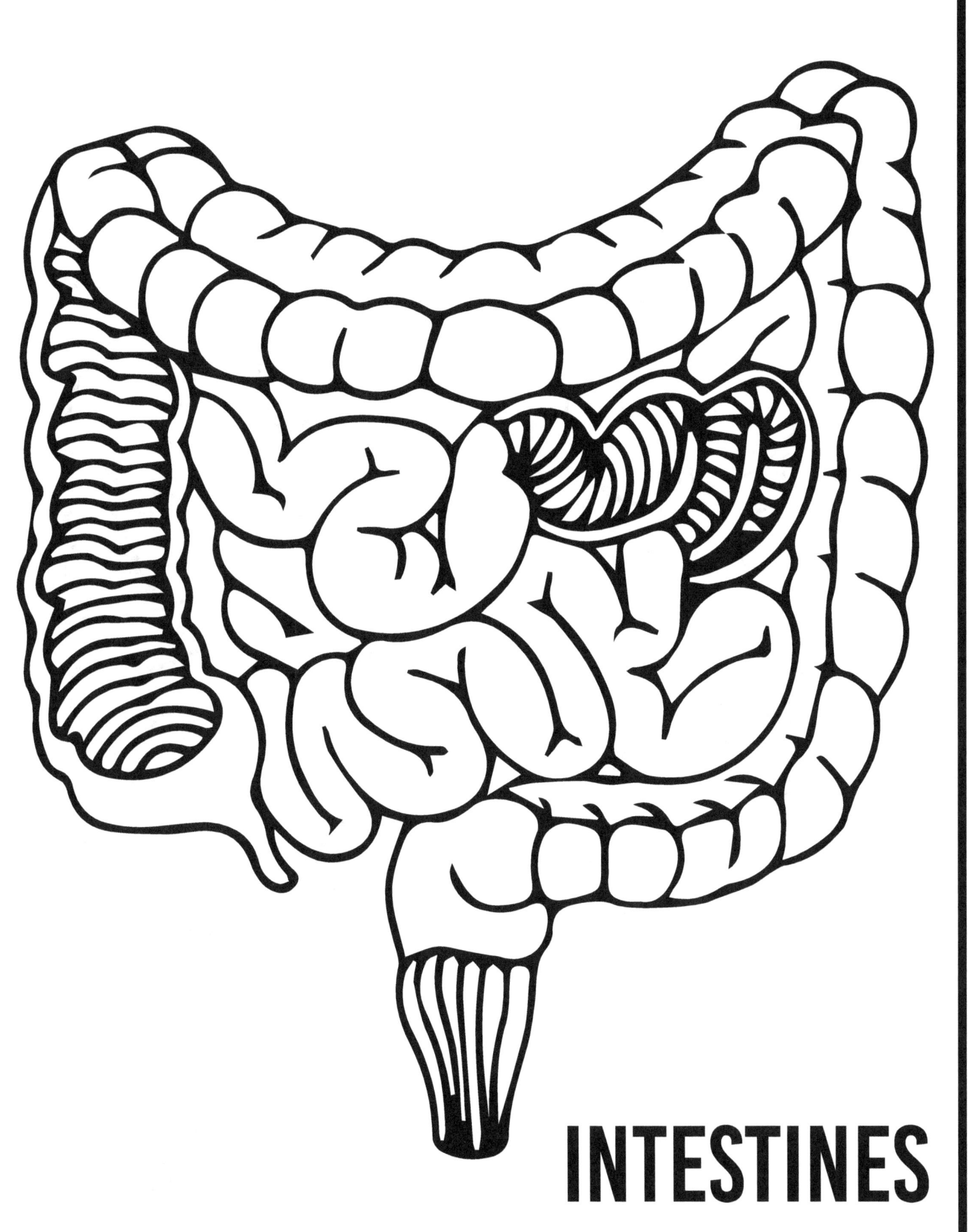

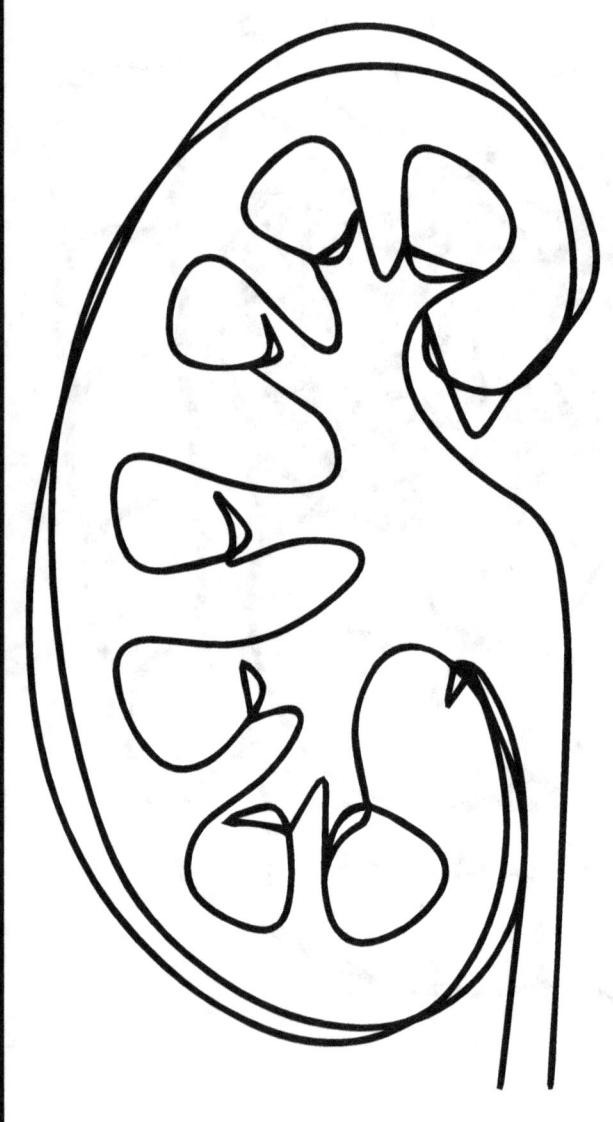
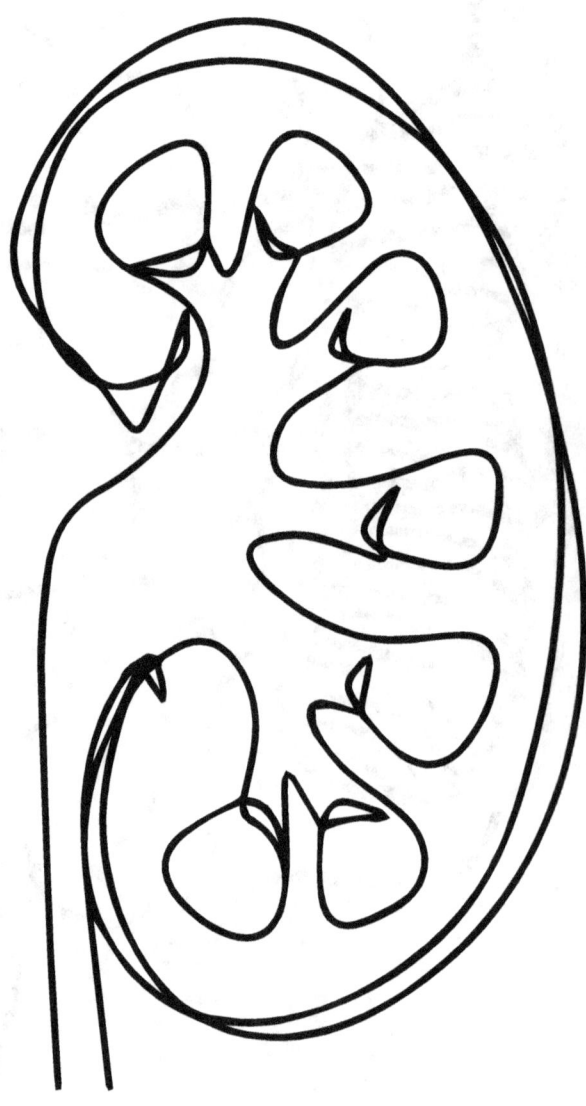

KIDNEYS

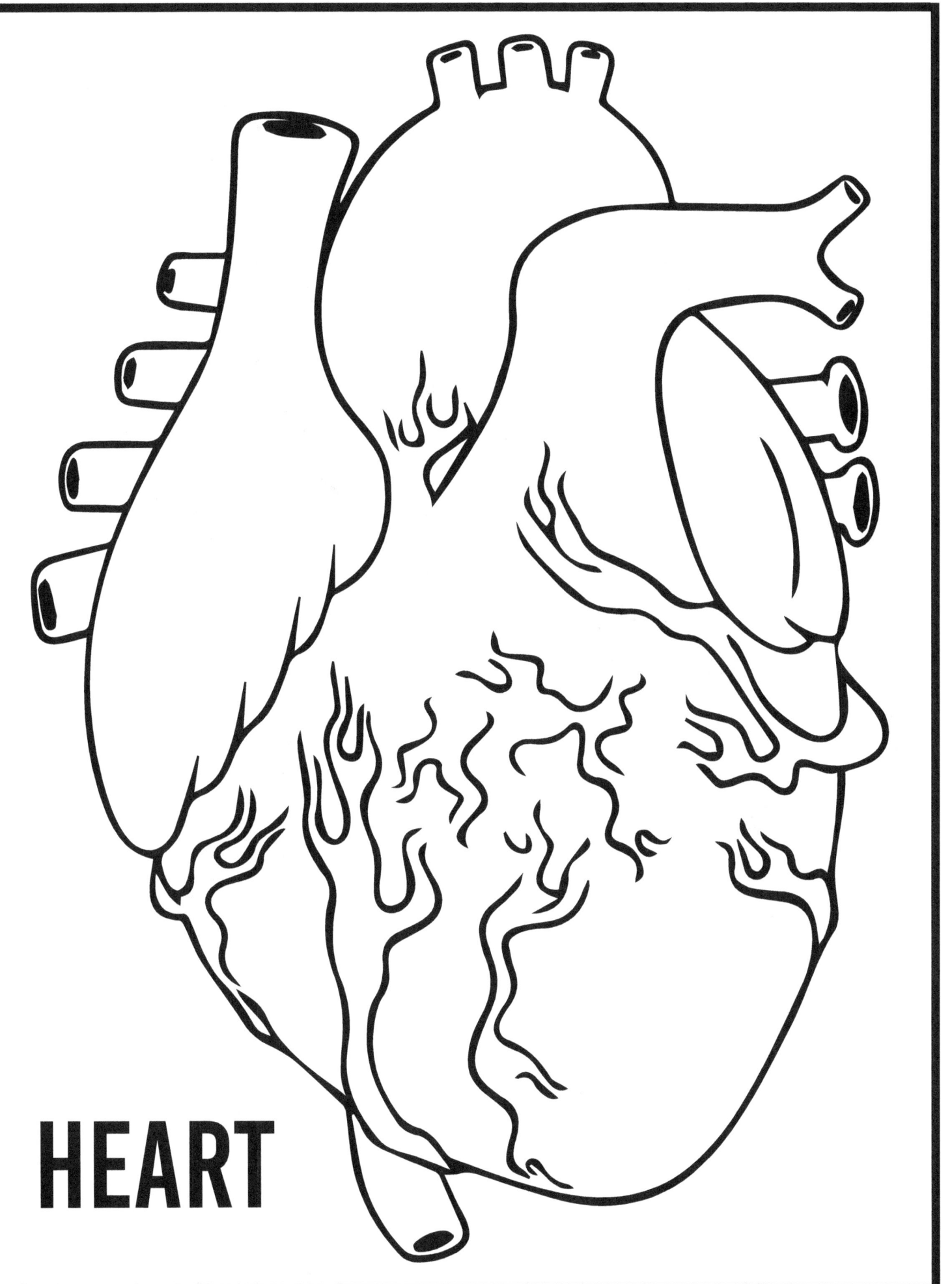

LUNGS

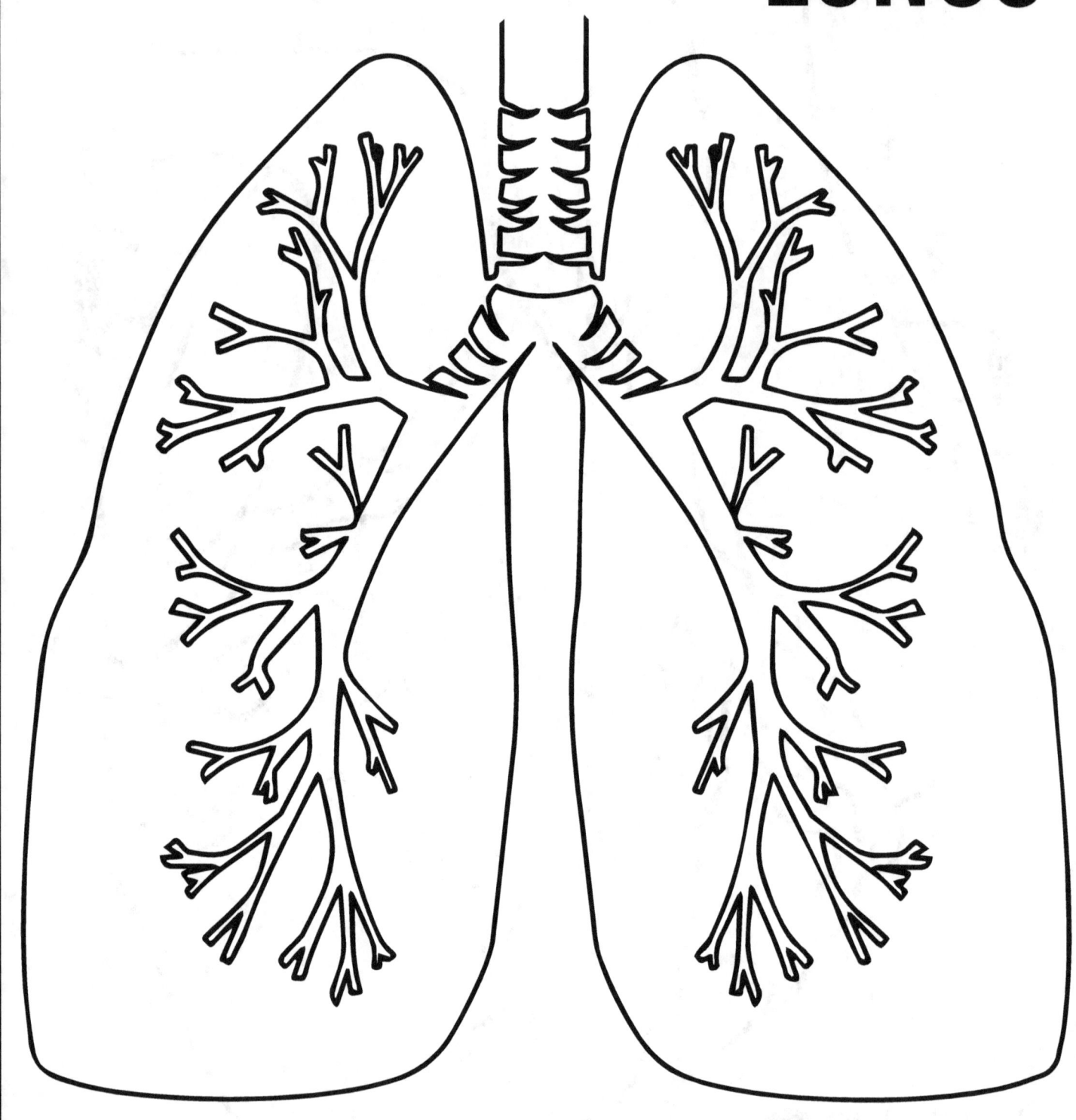

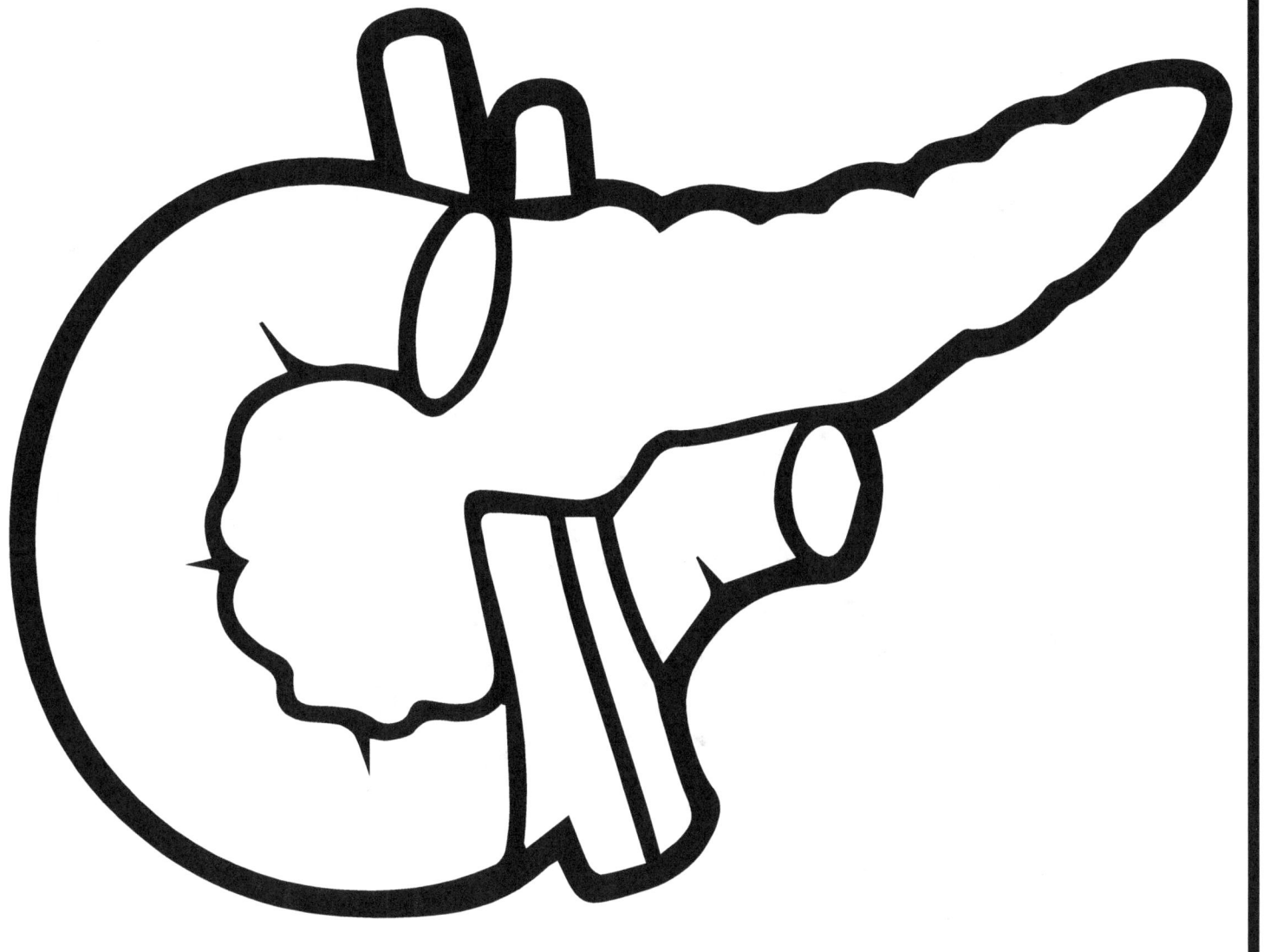

PANCREAS

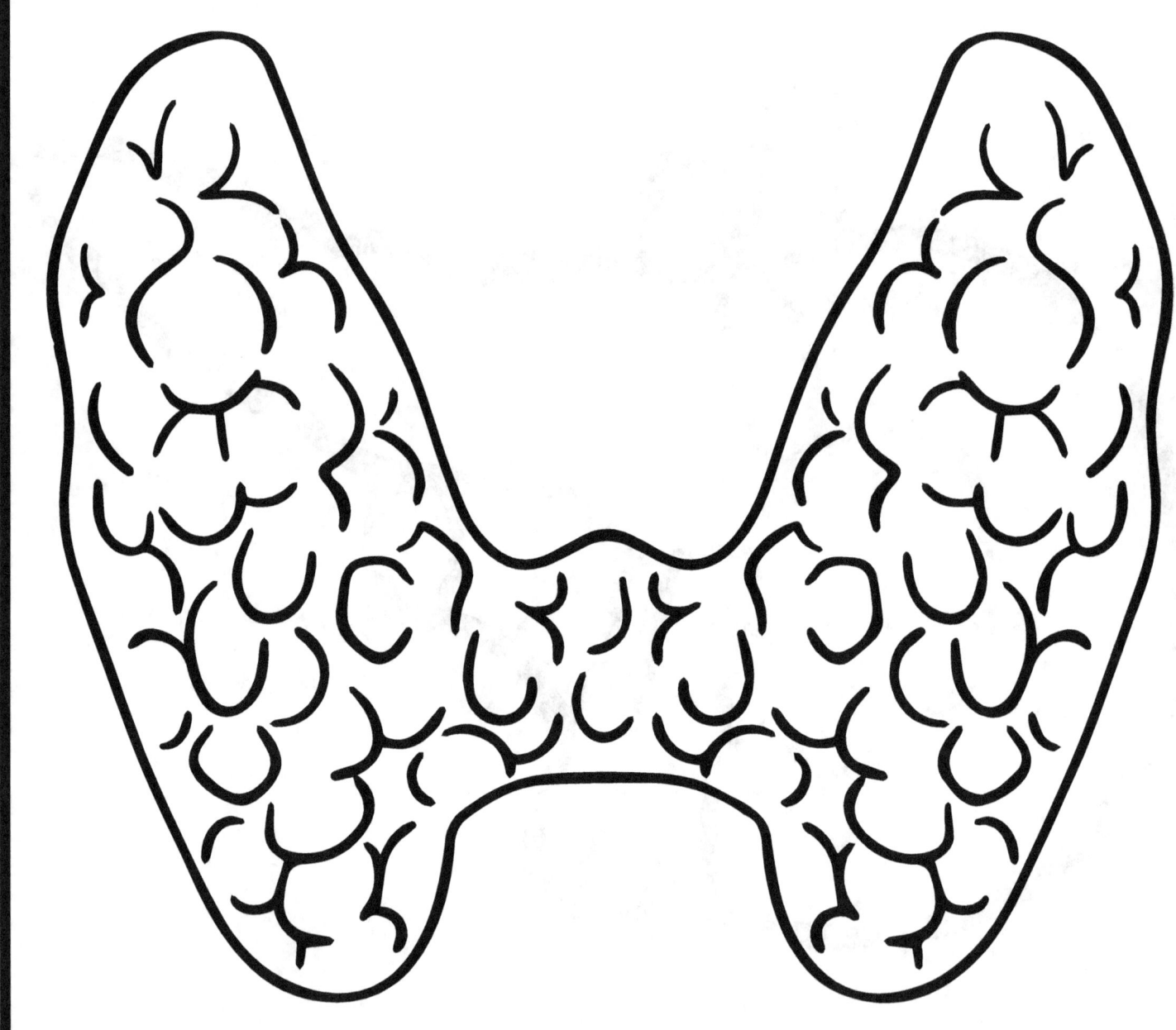

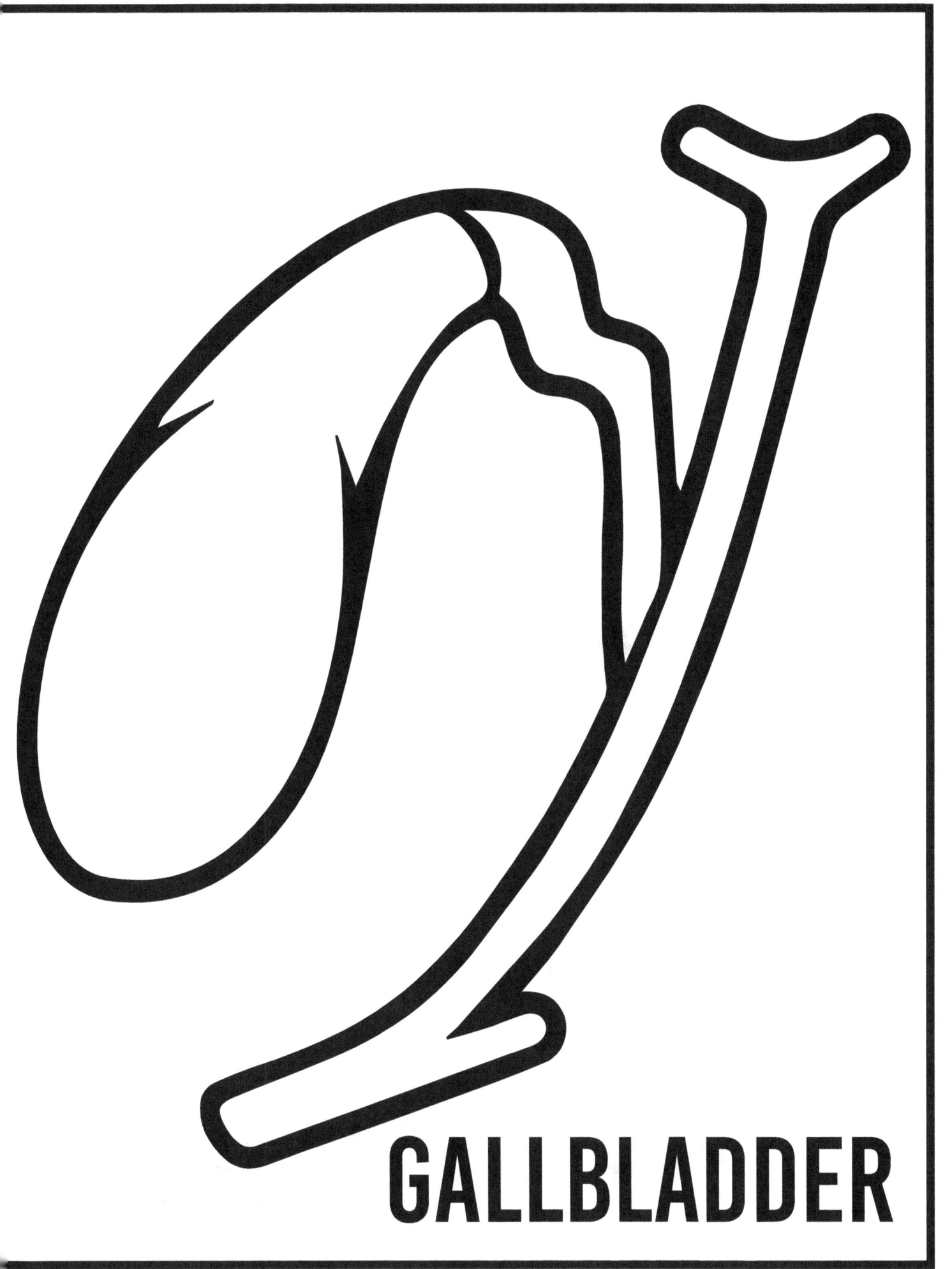

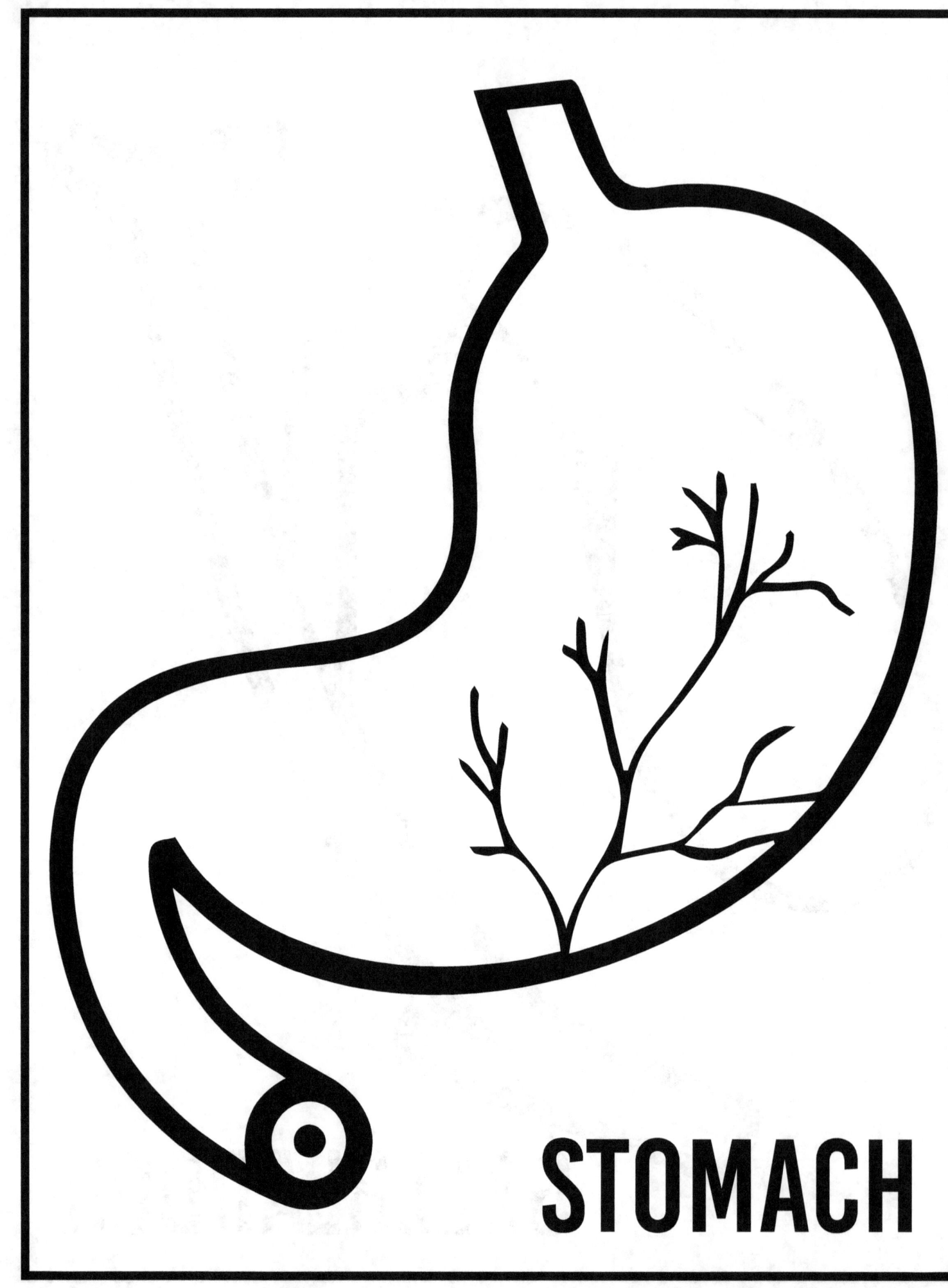

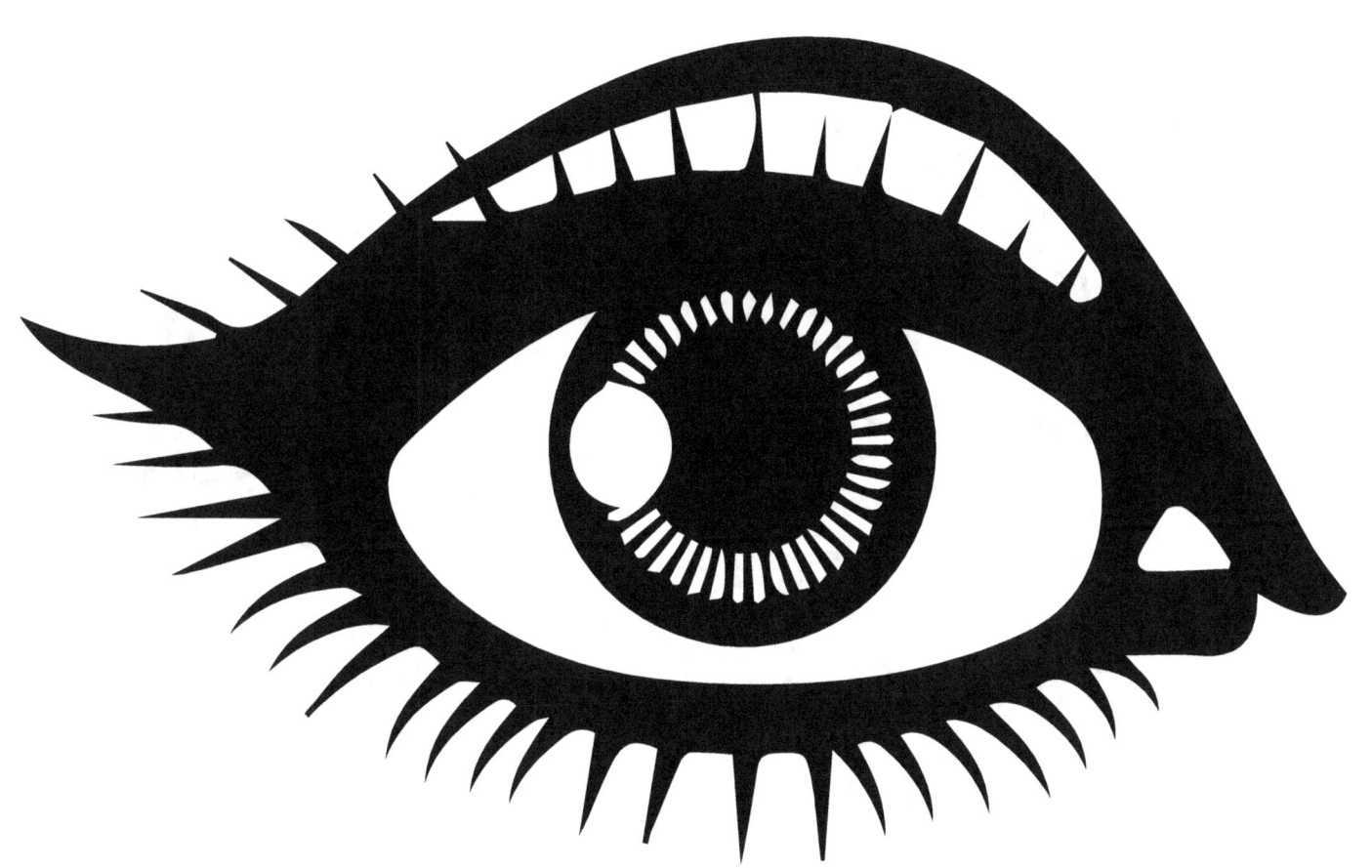

EYE

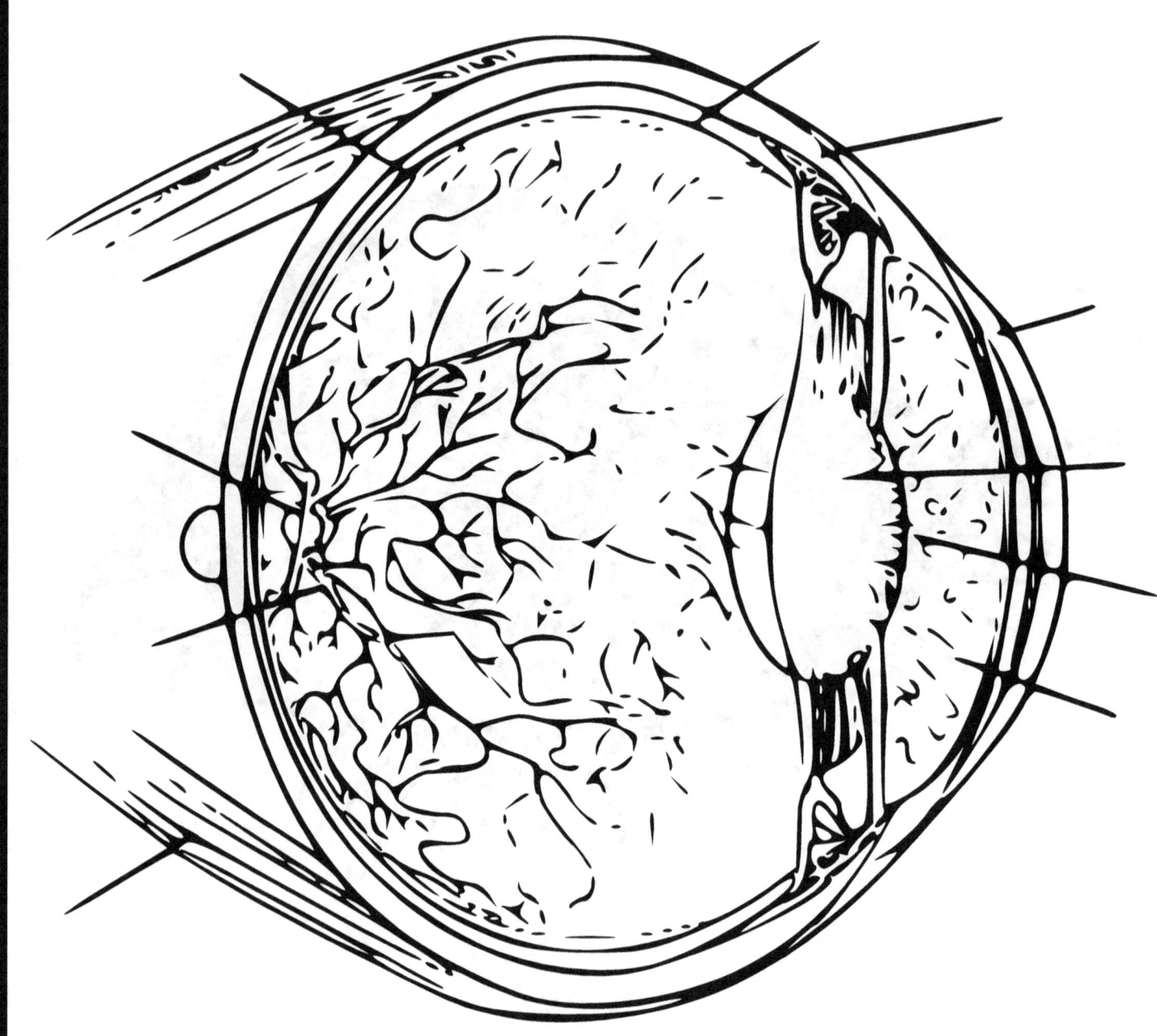

EYE (CROSS-SECTION)

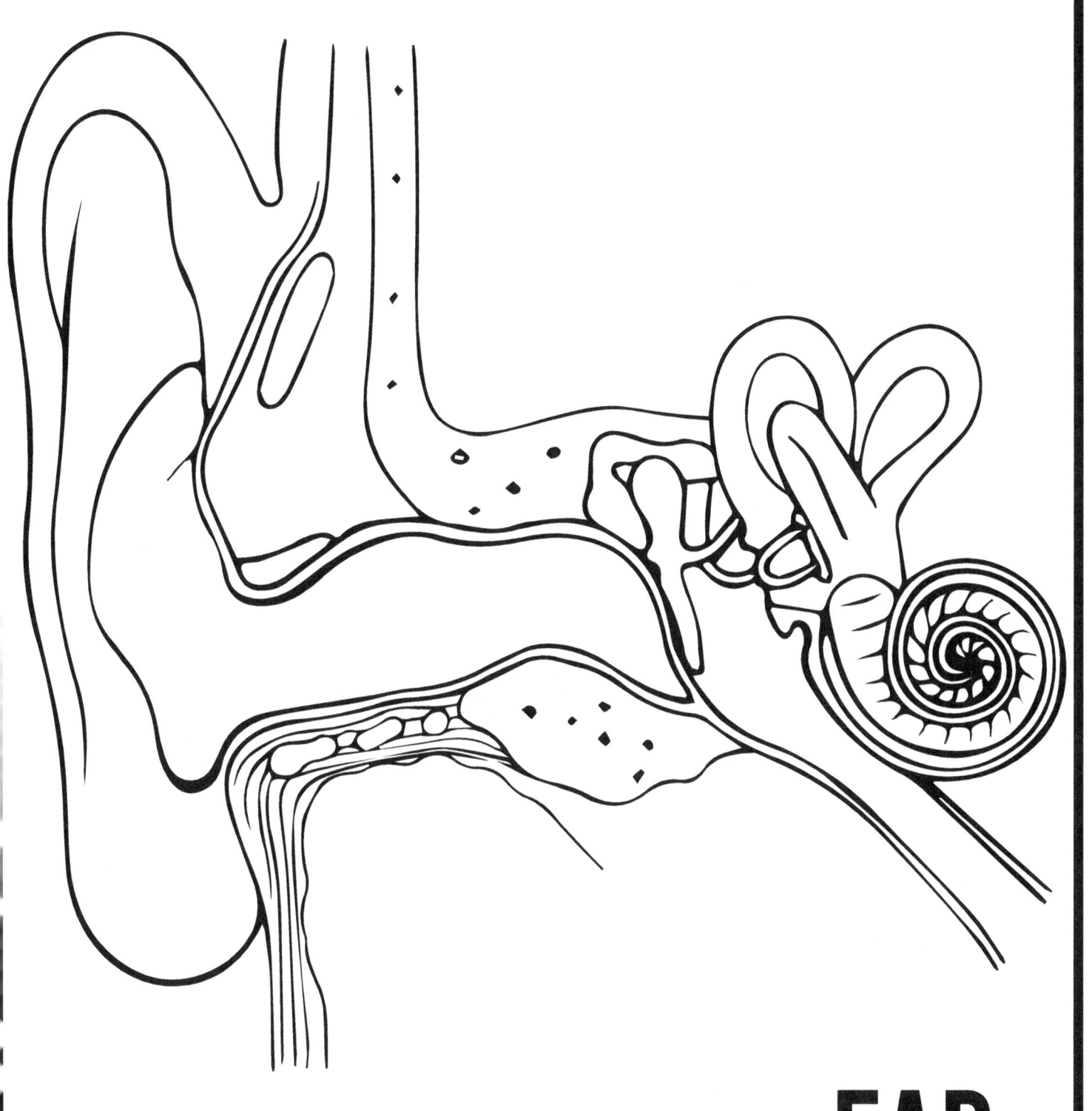

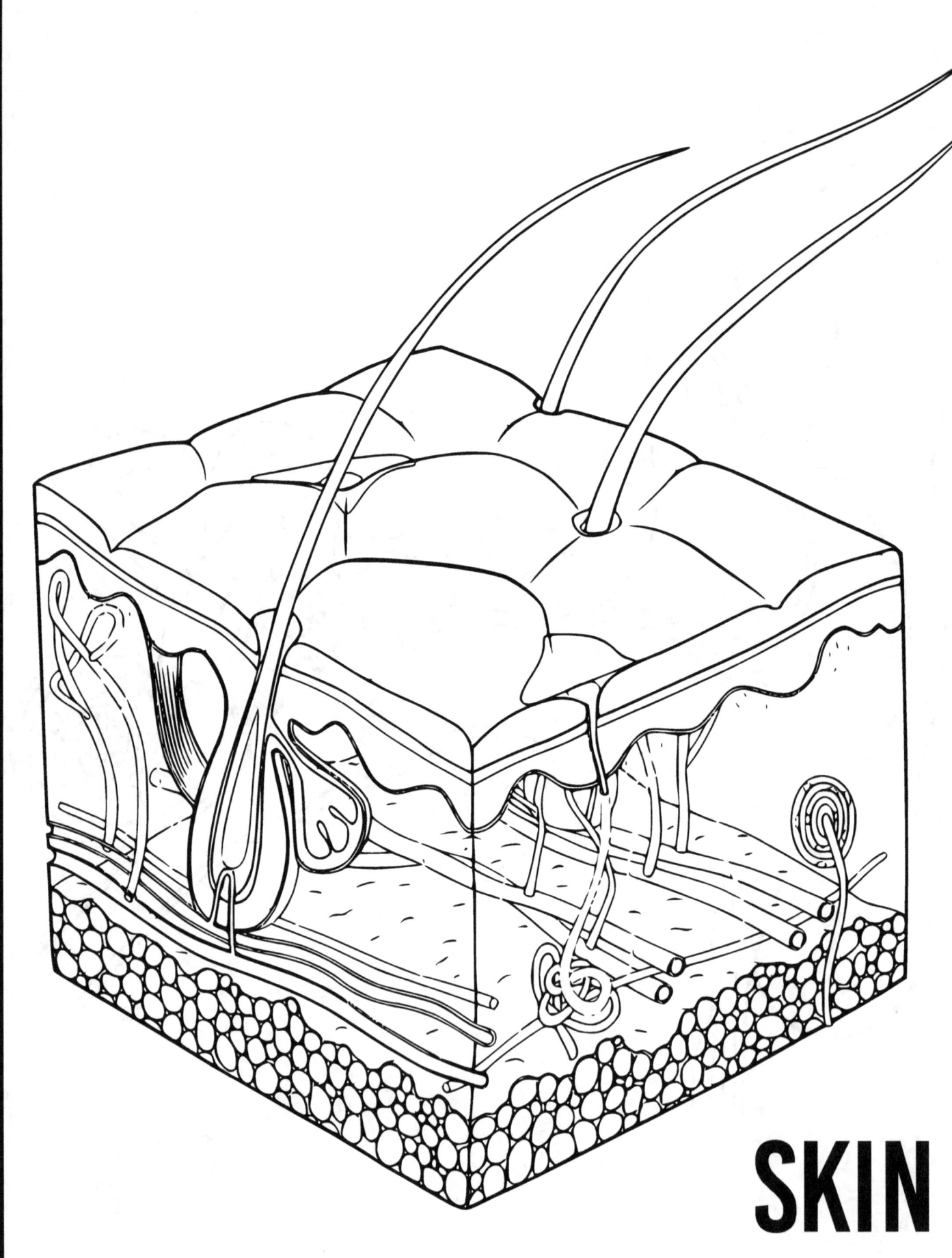

SKIN

TONGUE

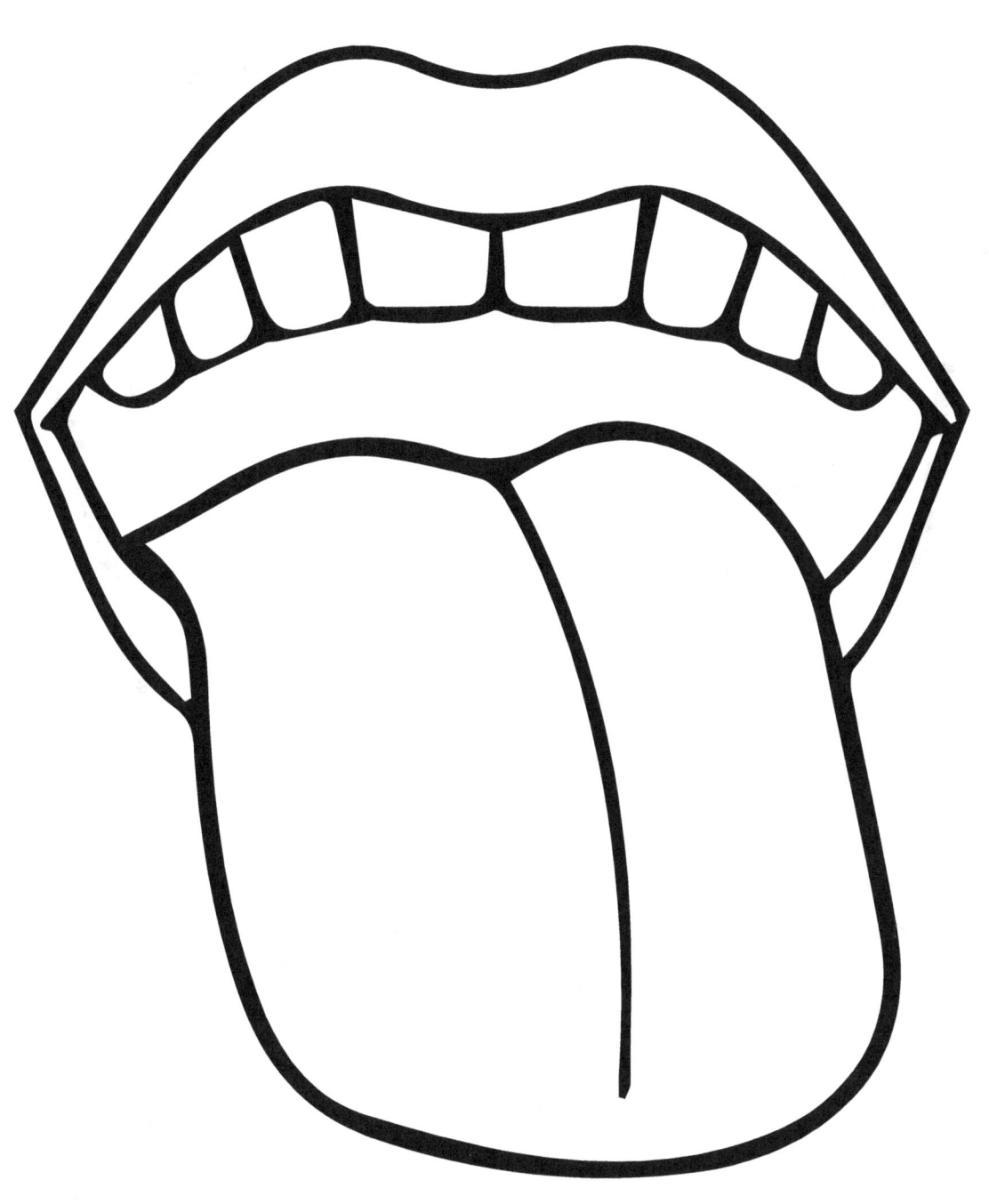

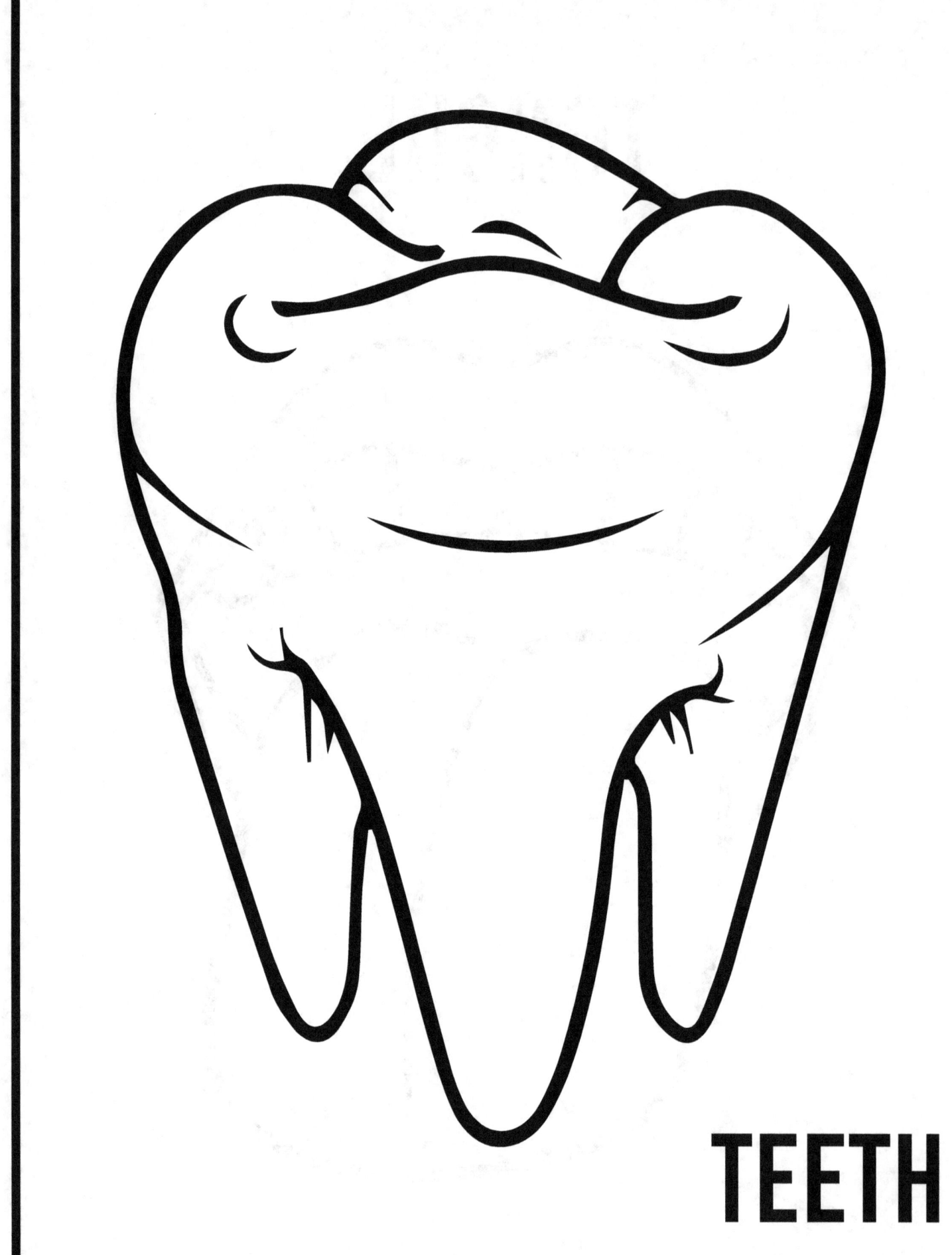

BLOOD CELLS

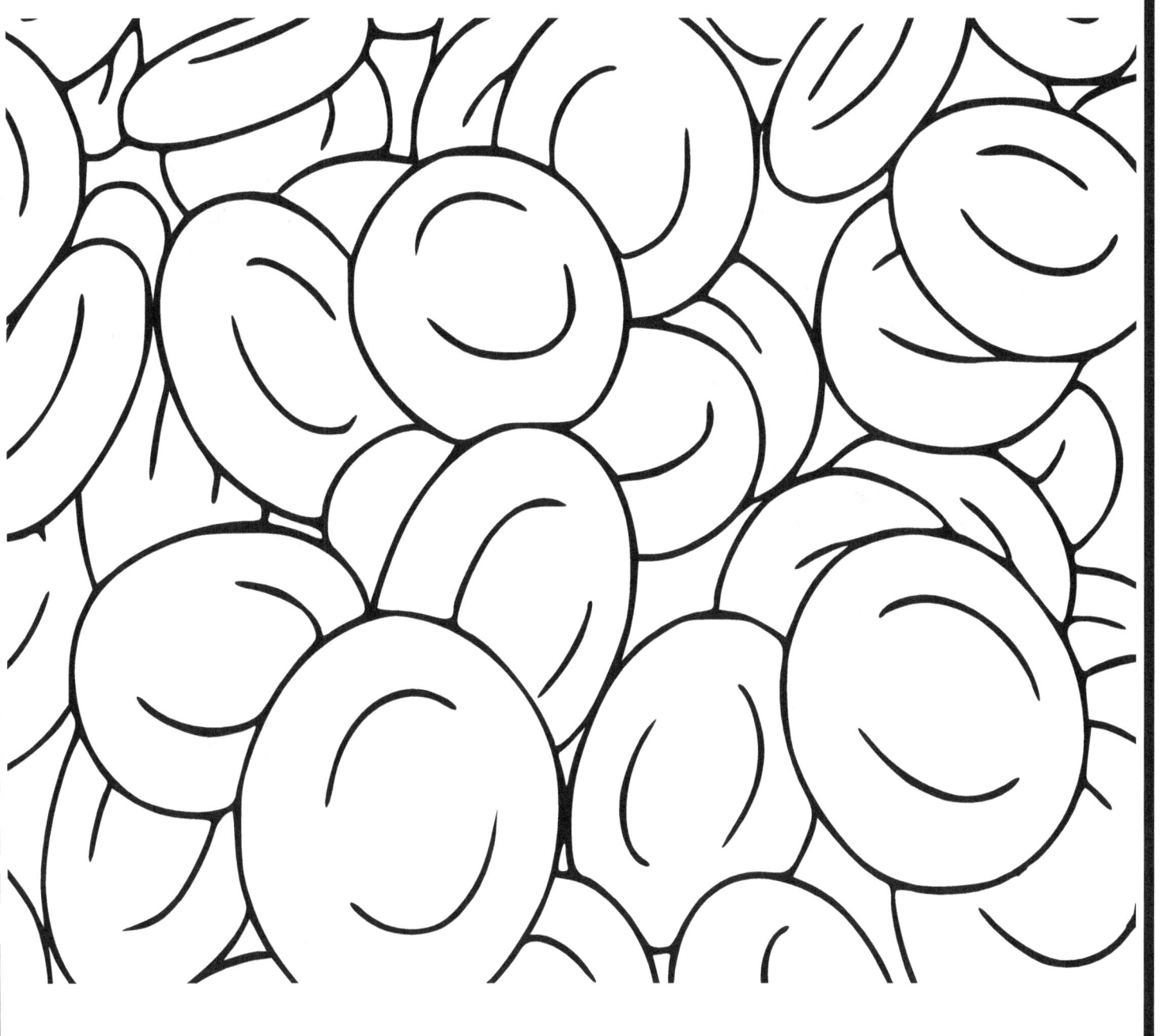

MUSCLE

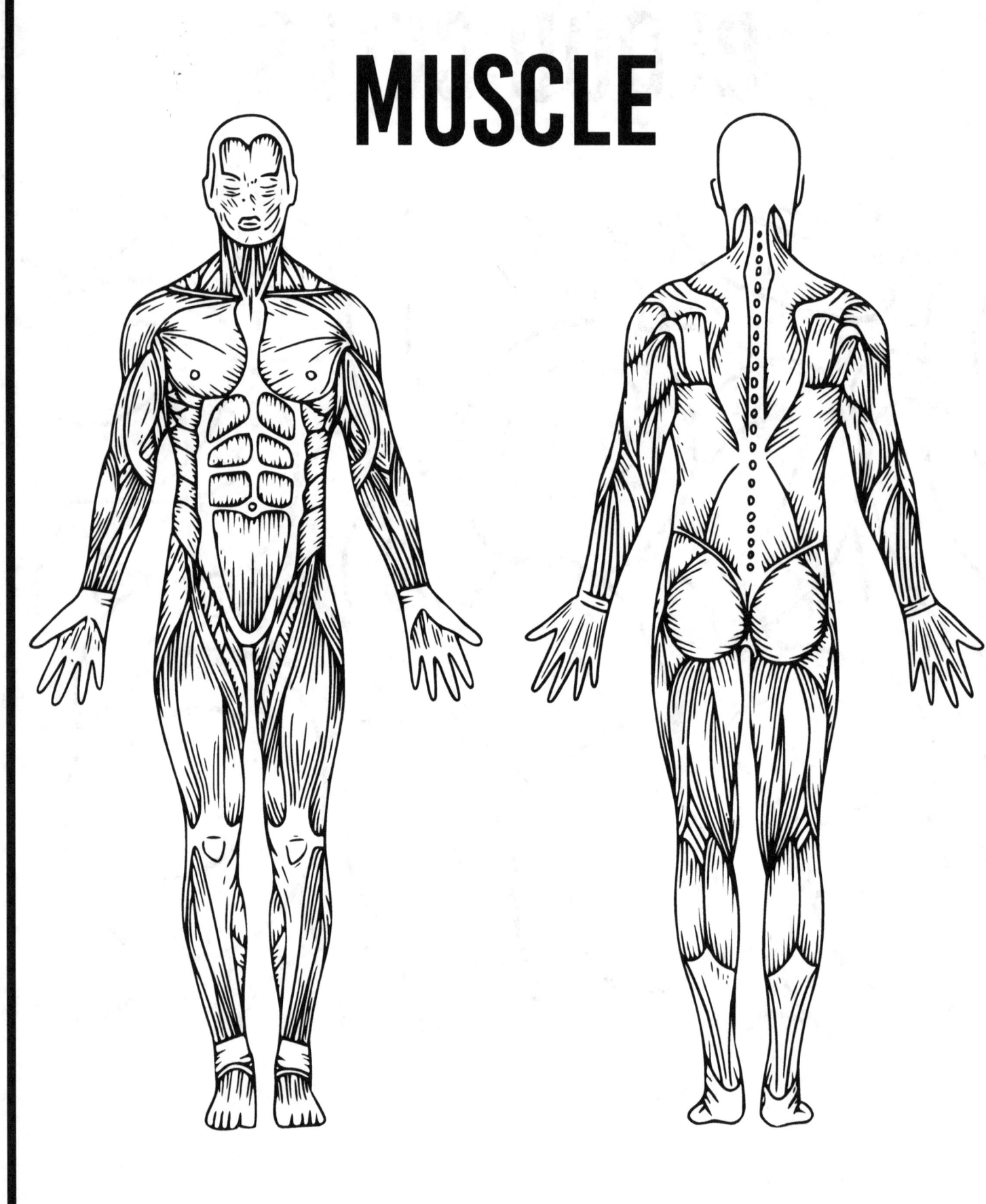

ARTERY

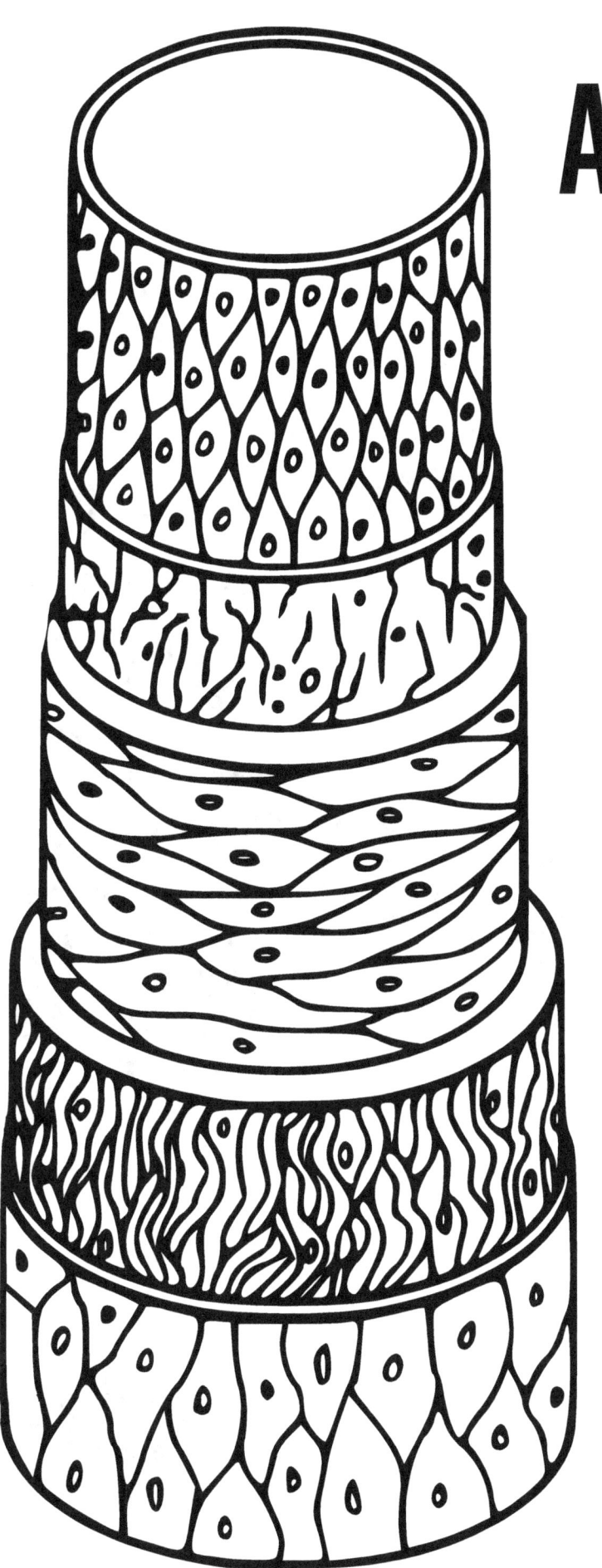

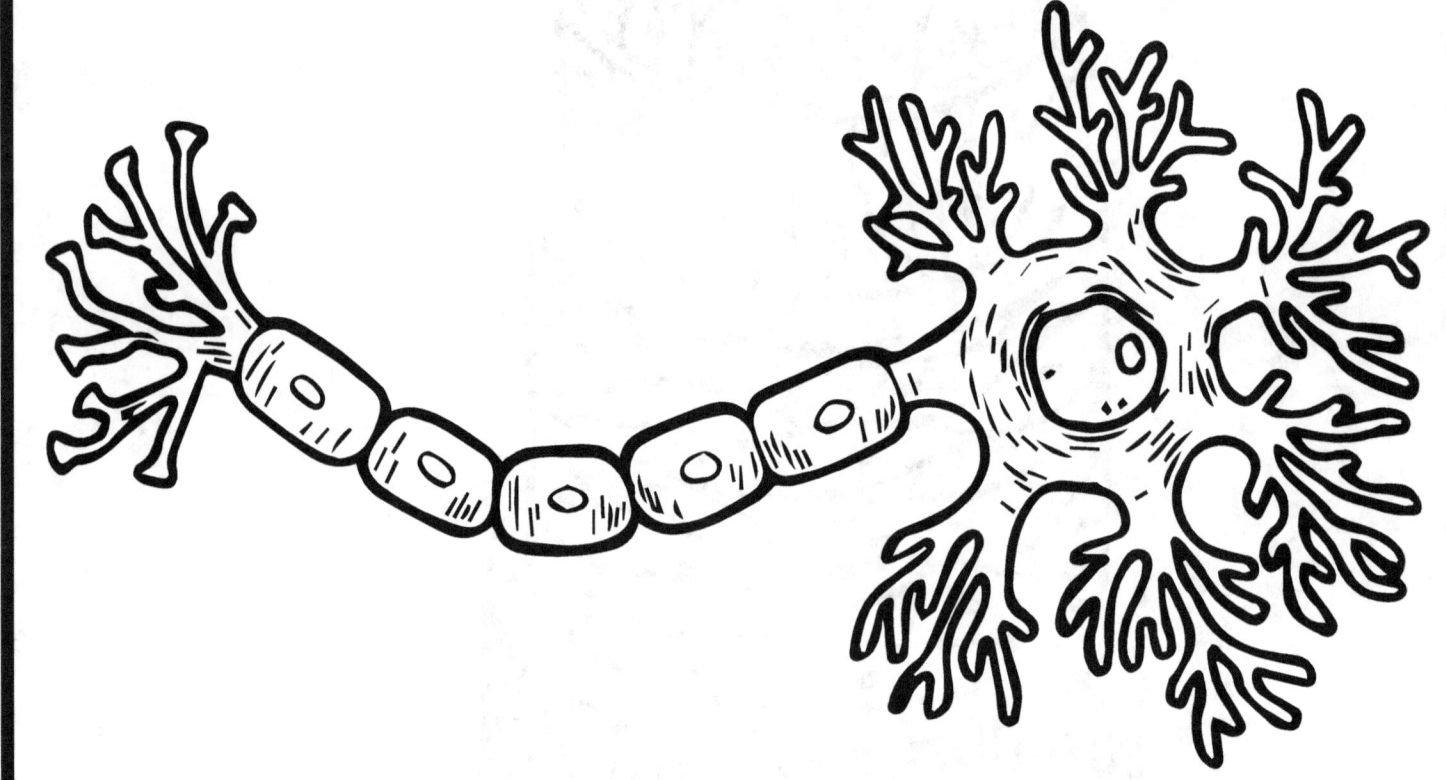

NEURON

www.ingramcontent.com/pod-product-compliance
Lightning Source LLC
Chambersburg PA
CBHW080817220526
45466CB00011BB/3599